PRAISE FOR

HEALING THE HUNGRY SELF

"Written with warmth, understanding, humor, and a feeling that the author really cares about those she is trying to help. . . . An invaluable addition to the effort to help those struggling with some of society's all-too-common problems."

—RONEE HERRMANN, M.D.,
Psychiatrist specializing in
eating-disorders treatment, Scarsdale, NY

"This interactive workbook offers a logical step-by-step approach that guides readers through the specific stages necessary to develop a healthy relationship with food and self. Practitioners and clients alike will benefit greatly from Dr. Price's experience, clinically acquired wisdom, and empathetic narrative style."

—DYANE LEMOS, PH.D.
Eating-disorders and weight-
management specialist,
San Diego, CA

DEIRDRA PRICE, Ph.D., President and CEO of Diet-Free Solution, is a licensed psychologist, speaker and seminar-leader, who conducts individual, group, and family therapy. She has facilitated groups for the National Association of Anorexia Nervosa and Associated Disorders, and has worked extensively in both in-patient and out-patient hospital-based eating-disorder programs. Dr. Price has a private practice in San Diego, California.

Here's to your good Health.

Deirdra Price

2007

HEALING THE HUNGRY SELF

The Diet-Free Solution to Lifelong Weight Management

DEIRDRA PRICE, Ph.D.

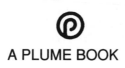

A PLUME BOOK

PLUME
Published by the Penguin Group
Penguin Putnam Inc., 375 Hudson Street,
New York, New York 10014, U.S.A.
Penguin Books Ltd, 27 Wrights Lane, London W8 5TZ, England
Penguin Books Australia Ltd, Ringwood, Victoria, Australia
Penguin Books Canada Ltd, 10 Alcorn Avenue, Toronto, Ontario,
Canada M4V 3B2
Penguin Books (N.Z.) Ltd, 182–190 Wairau Road, Auckland 10,
New Zealand

Penguin Books Ltd, Registered Offices:
Harmondsworth, Middlesex, England

Published by Plume, an imprint of Dutton Signet,
a member of Penguin Putnam Inc.
Previously published by Diet Free Solution, Inc.

First Plume Printing, January, 1998
10 9 8 7 6 5 4 3 2

Library of Congress Cataloging-in-Publication Data
Price, Deirdra.
    Healing the hungry self, the diet-free solution to lifelong weight
management / Deirdra Price.
        p.   cm.
    Includes bibliographical references.
    ISBN 0-452-27940-2
        1. Eating disorders—Popular works. 2. Self-help techniques.
    3. Weight loss—Psychological aspects. 4. Food habits—Psychological
aspects. I. Title.
    [RC552. E18P75 1998]   97-29000
    616.85'26—dc21   CIP

Printed in the United States of America

To my husband, Farhad, my parents, John and Marcia, my siblings, Steven and Jennifer, and my grandparents, Dean and Mabel, who always believed in me.

CONTENTS

INTRODUCTION

Dear Reader:

If you struggle with food, weight, body image, or self-acceptance, then *Healing the Hungry Self* is for you. It doesn't matter if you are male or female, fat or thin. This book offers a balanced, diet-free solution to lifelong weight management. Whether you starve yourself to lose weight rapidly, binge uncontrollably on large amounts of food, purge to prevent weight gain, or graze incessantly throughout the day, *Healing the Hungry Self* can help. It provides principles and tools to alter the way you think about and deal with food. You'll create permanent changes in your weight—naturally. Your body will decide what it needs to weigh to be healthy. This book focuses on the physical, emotional, mental, and spiritual issues surrounding food so you understand not only *how* you use food but also *why* you turn to it for comfort, companionship, or consolation.

Healing the Hungry Self offers practical information and strategies to break away from the diet mentality and obsession with food and appearance. You learn how to eat and exercise in moderation so that you never have to deprive yourself of food again. This book helps you understand the emotional and mental issues that cause you to use food in unhealthy ways. And you will learn to develop and honor your spiritual side, knowing that you are not alone and that it's possible to listen to the messages of your soul—the deepest part of you that has the answers to your peace of mind. With this balanced approach, you'll be able to eat a variety of foods—more than you ever thought possible—and not gain weight. Best of all, you'll finally feel good about yourself.

The most important part of achieving success with food and weight-control issues is addressing the *whole* self. The title of this book, *Healing the Hungry Self,* refers to the whole self that hungers for more than food—in fact, that feels starved for love. All of us want to experience self-love, and love for and from others, which brings a sense of fulfillment, purpose, and worth. When love isn't available, many people substitute food.

Using this book, you'll learn how to develop self-acceptance—the first step in achieving self-love. Self-acceptance comes from holding realistic and positive beliefs about one's self, effectively managing a wide array of emotional experiences, and engaging in eating behaviors that are healthy and balanced. You'll discover that when you change your beliefs, you'll make very different kinds of choices. And, if you make different choices, your beliefs are powerfully affected and altered.

For example, say you believe, "Eating chocolate cake will make me fat." After reading this book, you will learn that eating chocolate cake in moderation will *not* make you fat. You will trust the information enough to test yourself. The next time you go out for dinner, choose to top off your meal with a rich piece of Dutch chocolate cake. If you follow the rules and eat only one piece, you'll be surprised over the next few days when your weight *doesn't* rise one ounce. With that experience, you can change your belief to "Eating chocolate cake in moderation will not make me fat, and, in fact, I can eat anything I want, within reason," which begins to make a big difference in how you live your life.

The focus on the whole self makes this program different from the others you've tried, and it will bring the results you desire. Plus *Healing the Hungry Self*'s workbook format will help you stop and think about what you're doing and why. The exercises provided allow you to rate and explore personal patterns and habits. They show you how to change your thinking and behavior. Worksheets allow you to chart successes and make changes at your own pace.

As a therapist with over ten years' experience treating patients who have weight-control problems and eating disorders, I have watched many people heal, meaning that their behaviors are no longer causing physical, emotional, or mental problems. In my experience, weight-control success comes from a step-by-step approach using a variety of strategies and techniques that address areas specific to weight-management problems. Learning how to alter negative beliefs, effectively deal with feelings and thoughts, develop self-acceptance, make specific changes in eating behaviors, and honor your spiritual side are the keys to your success.

If you struggle with food, weight, body image, and self-acceptance, there is hope. You have the capability to heal, and this workbook will provide you with a wide variety of tools to aid you in the process—and they really work! I trust that you will choose to use them, since you deserve to be as happy and healthy as you can possibly be.

Please take good care of yourself. Make a daily commitment to heal and you will soon see positive changes. Here's to a happier and healthier you!

Deirdra Price, Ph.D.

HOW TO USE THE WORKBOOK: THE SIX-WEEK PLAN

By completing one chapter of this workbook per day, you can accomplish the *Diet-Free Solution* in six weeks. The most important factor is to work at a pace that's comfortable for you—something only you can decide. Take as long as you need to get the full benefit from the advice offered.

Some people read a chapter a day and do the accompanying exercises. Others find it more helpful to read a chapter and to begin implementing changes in their lives before moving on to the next chapter. I recommend that you read each chapter and complete the exercises in the order in which they are presented. However, you may want to skip chapters that are not applicable to you or to read only those chapters that offer help for what you're needing to work on right now.

Each chapter is assigned a day, which you'll find on top of the first page. After you read the chapter, there's an assignment for you to complete. Each assignment consists of assessing and analyzing your behaviors, thoughts, feelings, and choices as they relate to how you deal with food, weight, body-image, and self-acceptance. You'll then fill out charts and finish worksheets that will help you make changes in each of these areas so that you become healthier physically, emotionally, mentally, and spiritually.

At the end of this chapter is a schedule to help you set up your plan of recovery. Use this schedule to set aside time for each chapter and to keep track of your progress and success.

Week 1 Overview

Read *1-2* to *1-5* in **Part One: Unhealthy Eating Behaviors** and fill out all the checklists. This will give you an idea of how your eating behaviors may be harming you and what physical, emotional, and mental symptoms you're currently experiencing. Awareness of what your body and mind are going through will give you the necessary input to begin applying the information in the upcoming chapters of the book. You'll then read chapters

2-1 and 2-2 of **Part Two: Healing the Physical Self** which describe the addictive nature of food-related disorders as well as why diets don't work and what really does work.

Week 2 Overview

Focus on changing your eating behaviors by reading chapters 2-3 to 2-9 and completing the accompanying worksheets in the rest of **Part Two: Healing the Physical Self.** The main goal is to plan your meals and eat three meals a day, with or without snacks. Notice what kinds of foods you gravitate toward, which foods you have trouble incorporating into your meal plans, what you crave and can't seem to live without, and which meals seem the easiest and hardest to eat on a consistent basis. You'll begin to see the difference between physical and emotional hunger and learn how to include forbidden foods into your meal plans. Don't expect to have mastered three meals a day in one week. By the end of week two, however, you will have the foundation to develop a habit of eating healthfully and moderately each day.

Week 3 Overview

Address your eating behaviors by building on what you learned last week. Read chapters 2-10 to 2-16 and complete the accompanying exercises in **Part Two: Healing the Physical Self.** You'll begin to include forbidden foods in your meal plans, reverse eating rituals, recognize danger zones, delay and eventually prevent harmful behaviors, set up an exercise plan, accept your body, use alternatives to food to cope with your emotions, and reduce the likelihood of relapsing into old, unhealthy patterns.

By the end of week three, you will be eating three meals a day, reducing unhealthy behaviors, performing some form of exercise, accepting yourself more, and using alternatives to food abuse. If you're overweight, you'll start to see weight loss, as long as you're not bingeing or grazing. If you're underweight, you'll begin to gain weight. Your weight will adjust itself naturally. Let your body set the pace.

Week 4 Overview

Begin the process of understanding your belief system, emotional experiences, and thought processes described in **Part Three: Healing the Emotional Self and the Mental Self.** With chapters 3-1 to 3-7, you'll explore your personal set of negative beliefs, attitudes, thoughts, and feelings, and how they affect your choices. You'll meet your child, adolescent, critic, and internal healer—all of whom have a part in reinforcing your unhealthy eating behaviors. In *Game 1—Distorted Thinking,* you'll see how your critical voice keeps you stuck in a cycle of unhealthy eating patterns by encouraging you to perceive your world negatively. You'll learn how to talk back to your critic to reduce the harsh internal dialogue and make way for more positive beliefs.

By the end of week four, you'll have strengthened your new eating behaviors by focusing daily on eating and exercising moderately. Weight loss or gain may continue or stabilize, depending on how your body reacts to the changes you've made. You'll have an understanding of the reasons underlying your unhealthy eating behaviors and, you'll be more in touch with your internal life, understanding how your history shaped you. You'll now have the tools to reduce your distorted thinking and quiet the critic within.

Week 5 Overview

Focus on the rest of the games in chapter *3-7* and then work on chapters *3-8* to *3-10* in **Part Three: Healing the Emotional Self and the Mental Self.** Set time aside to read about the games you play with yourself and to complete the accompanying worksheets. Notice the close relationship between unresolved issues and eating behaviors. As you deal with the underlying reasons of why you approach food in the way you do, your eating patterns will become healthier. Now, it's time to create affirmations that will allow you to accept your flaws and stop rejecting yourself. You'll also learn how to relax and bust stress. Use visualizations to change your beliefs. You alter beliefs by healing shame and pain, rewriting your beliefs in your head, or giving back a belief—with the accompanying thoughts and feelings—to the person who originally gave it to you.

By the end of week five, your new eating behavior will be much more of a habit—more automatic. Some areas may be more difficult to master and may take more time. You'll experience more body acceptance and be gentler with yourself. You'll be actively working with your critical voice and negative beliefs to reduce them. You're now conscious of what your issues are and you'll have the tools to address them.

Week 6 Overview

Finally, focus on developing your spiritual self in **Part Four: Healing the Spiritual Self.** Take time to get in touch with your soul and to define what spirituality means to you. This process will help you create a sense of meaning in your life. **Part Five: Conclusion** will help you continue to attend to your eating behaviors and to work through whatever issues remain. There's a chapter for addressing family members' concerns. With this workbook, you'll have the tools to face any remaining issues.

Follow these guidelines to help you use this workbook effectively. Remember, you decide the pace that's comfortable for you. These are only suggestions, not the law. Use whatever information is helpful, and return to it as often as necessary to alter the way you think about and deal with food, weight, and body-image. You have whatever it takes to make the necessary changes. You can do it!

SIX-WEEK PLAN SCHEDULE

Fill in the date and check (✓) the chapters you finished reading and the assignments you have completed. Use this schedule to keep you on track and to assess your progress and success.

WEEK 1

DAY	CHAPTER	DATE	READING	ASSIGNMENT
1	1-1 Choose to Heal			
2	1-2 Your Many Selves			
3	1-3 Warning! How You Eat Can Harm You			
4	1-4 The Body Factor			
5	1-5 Your Heart and Head			
6	2-1 Why Do I Keep Doing This?			
7	2-2 Diets Make You Fatter			

WEEK 2

DAY	CHAPTER	DATE	READING	ASSIGNMENT
1	2-3 Three Meals a Day Keep the Weight Away			
2	2-4 Knock Down Barriers to Success			
3	2-5 Reduce the Food Obsession			
4	2-6 Meals Made Easy			
5	2-7 Chart Your Way to Change			
6	2-8 Physical Hunger vs. Emotional Hunger			
7	2-9 Bust the "Bad" Foods Myth			

WEEK 3

DAY	CHAPTER	DATE	READING	ASSIGNMENT
1	2-10 Reverse Eating Rituals			
2	2-11 Recognize Your Danger Zones			
3	2-12 Frequency, Quantity, Quality			
4	2-13 Get Moving!			
5	2-14 Stop Body Hate			
6	2-15 Face Your Feelings			
7	2-16 Relapse			

WEEK 4

DAY	CHAPTER	DATE	READING	ASSIGNMENT
1	*3-1 From Here to There*			
2	*3-2 Understanding Your Crutch*			
3	*3-3 The Power of Negative Beliefs*			
4	*3-4 Your Players*			
5	*3-5 You Are What You Believe*			
6	*3-6 How You Feel and Think*			
7	*3-7 The Mind Games; Game 1—Distorted Thinking*			

WEEK 5

DAY	CHAPTER	DATE	READING	ASSIGNMENT
1	*Game 2—Perfectionism*			
2	*Game 3—Watchful Eye*			
3	*Game 4—Nonassertiveness*			
4	*Game 5—Anticipation*			
5	*3-8 Affirm Yourself Daily*			
6	*3-9 Progressive Relaxation*			
7	*3-10 Visualizations That Alter Beliefs*			

WEEK 6

DAY	CHAPTER	DATE	READING	ASSIGNMENT
1	*4-1 Tending to the Soul*			
2	*5-1 On the Path to Recovery*			
3	*5-2 A New Lifestyle*			
4	*5-3 For the Family*			
5	*5-4 Reap Success*			

PART ONE:
UNHEALTHY
EATING
BEHAVIORS

1 - 1

Choose to Heal:
It's Finally Time to Love Yourself

Each year approximately 44 million people try to lose weight, spending $30 billion on diet foods, pills, and special regimens. Yet 90 to 95 percent of those who lose weight fail

---

*"In spite of all the diet information available,
Americans keep getting heavier as time goes on."*

---

to keep it off and often gain back more than they lost. In spite of all the diet information available, Americans keep getting heavier as time goes on. A record 71 percent of people ages 25 and older are considered overweight today, compared with 69 percent in 1994 and 56 percent in 1984. Another eight million people deliberately starve themselves or alternately binge eat and purge in an attempt to reach an ideal appearance.

Striving to meet narrow social standards of beauty leads hundreds of thousands of people each year to learn to dislike their bodies. In misguided efforts to change their appearance, they develop unhealthy, and often downright dangerous eating habits—ranging from deprivation and starvation to bingeing and purging, or perpetually grazing on unhealthy foods.

If you're caught on this roller coaster ride, it's time to get off. Whether you're normal weight, underweight, or five, fifty, or a hundred pounds overweight, if you struggle with food, weight control, body image, and self-acceptance problems, *Healing the Hungry Self* offers you a diet-free solution. It will help you determine *why* you eat, giving you the understanding you need to work on the behaviors that cause the compulsion. When you change negative beliefs, manage your emotions, learn new behaviors, and honor your spirit, your body will weigh a healthy weight. You will like yourself—even love yourself—and be free of the obsession once and for all.

Developing self-acceptance and self-love includes knowing how to nurture and take care of physical needs like eating, sleeping, grooming, and exercise. It also means building a confident sense of self based on positive and realistic beliefs and allowing yourself to experience a wide variety of emotions with relative comfort and ease. Self-acceptance also means developing body wisdom—letting your body decide what it needs to weigh to be healthy. Honoring your spiritual side is another ingredient in the self-love recipe. When you can experience love for yourself, you can then give and receive love more easily because you open the door for these kinds of experiences.

"You can experience problems similar to those of someone who has an eating disorder without actually having the full-blown symptoms of the disorder yourself."

When you don't feel self-love, it's easy to neglect yourself. You probably had negative perceptions about yourself before your unhealthy eating behaviors began. Now, engaging in these behaviors perpetuates your feelings that you're unlovable, imperfect, stupid, weak, and generally a "mess." Problems with food often lead to feelings of helplessness and hopelessness. Yet, sneaking a bowl of ice cream smothered in chocolate fudge after everyone has gone to bed may be so much a part of your evening ritual that you can't imagine living without the midnight fix. Unhealthy patterns like this become a coping mechanism for many painful feelings that are fueled by negative beliefs about yourself. Unpleasant emotions can drive you to eat.

At the far end of the spectrum, extreme eating behaviors fit the criteria for *anorexia nervosa*, *bulimia nervosa*, or *binge eating disorder* (compulsive overeating). However, you can experience problems similar to those of someone who has an eating disorder without actually having the full-blown symptoms of the disorder yourself. With an actual disorder, the symptoms are simply more pronounced. The level of distress, however, can be the same. You will want to take advantage of the techniques in this workbook if you have any of the following signs:

- Constantly think about food throughout the day

- Eat when you're not hungry but don't know why

- Eat when stressed out, bored, anxious, depressed, angry, or lonely

- Have tried every diet and exercise program on the market

- Continue to diet even though it doesn't lead to permanent weight loss

- Feel concerned or depressed about your weight, shape, and appearance

- Find that your happiness depends on what you weigh and how you look

- "Feel fat" and limit your activities as a result

- Greatly dislike your body and consider taking extreme measures to change it

- Engage in vigorous, long, and often painful exercise workouts to lose weight

- Think about purging (vomiting, laxatives, diuretics, excessive exercise) but have never followed through

- Engage in vomiting, use enemas, exercise excessively, or take laxatives, diuretics, diet pills, cocaine, crack, speed, or ephedrine to keep off weight

- Starve yourself as a way to control weight

- Have episodes of eating large amounts of food, vowing afterward to never do it again

The emotional issues and the behavioral patterns are similar across the range of unhealthy eating styles, and this workbook will help you address all the areas you need to work on to become healthier—physically, emotionally, mentally, and spiritually.

Assignment: Identify individual signs that reflect your unhealthy relationship with food. Understand that your quest to be thin was an attempt to feel good about yourself. That's what *Healing the Hungry Self* is all about, developing healthy self-acceptance and self-love.

1 - 2

Your Many Selves:
How This Workbook Can Help You Recover
Physically, Emotionally, Mentally, and Spiritually

This workbook is specifically designed to focus on four important areas of the healing process: the physical self, the emotional self, the mental self, and the spiritual self. These areas are intimately and intricately linked together. However, for the sake of understanding how each operates and how to make specific changes in each area, I have divided them as if they function separately. They don't. Who you are is defined by an integrated self made up of the physical body, beliefs and thought processes, emotional experiences, and a spirit/soul connection.

I have separated all the selves because for many people, creating changes in the physical self is easier and usually comes before addressing emotional, mental, or spiritual issues. Others may feel more comfortable focusing on the emotional and mental aspects first and altering eating behaviors later. Still others need a spiritual basis from which to address every issue. Ultimately, all areas need to be addressed if change is to be successful and permanent. You can work on one area at a time, all areas simultaneously, or alternate between them. Within the four areas, eight specific changes are necessary for healing to occur. Each of these is addressed in the workbook.

These changes are:

1. Giving up dieting

2. Stopping unhealthy or destructive behaviors (i.e., purging)

3. Learning to eat three meals a day, with or without snacks

4. Maximizing the benefits of exercise while minimizing injury or burnout

5. Coping with feelings

6. Changing negative beliefs

7. Accepting yourself the way you are today

8. Honoring your spirit

Healing requires that you make a daily commitment to the process of change. Some days you must focus moment-to-moment on how you deal with food and what you're feeling and thinking. Other days will require less of your attention. Each day builds on the previous one, however, and eventually you'll establish new behavioral and thought patterns. Creating a habit takes a minimum of 21 days. After six weeks, the habit is strengthened and more difficult to break.

One of the most valuable ways to change your behaviors is to keep track of them. This workbook provides many opportunities for charting behaviors, feelings, and thoughts. I recommend you photocopy the charts you anticipate using often.

The workbook is divided into five chapters. The first describes unhealthy eating patterns, the second addresses behavioral changes you will need to make, the third focuses on the emotional and mental issues you will need to work through, the fourth addresses your spiritual condition, and the fifth discusses ways you can continue the healing process and maintain positive changes.

As you begin the process, while you're still engaging in unhealthy eating patterns, it's important to seek regular physical checkups, preferably with a physician who understands the specific medical problems associated with weight-management problems and food-related disorders.

Also, *Healing the Hungry Self* can be a valuable addition to ongoing individual psychotherapy and support groups. You may find it necessary to seek out one or both of these forms of therapy during the healing process. The more information, support, and help you can get, the easier the healing process will be. Nutritional counseling can help you learn about the nutritional value of different foods, portion sizes, and overall healthy eating.

The healing process can be difficult, yet exciting. This workbook provides you with the information and tools to make the necessary changes to free yourself from food, weight, and body-image issues. You *can* do it. Give yourself the time, permission, and commitment to heal. It can happen!

Assignment: Learn how this workbook can help you make changes in the eight essential areas of your life necessary for a complete recovery. Think about the changes you'll need to make in order to heal your unhealthy relationship with food.

1 - 3

Warning! How You Eat Can Harm You: Four Hazardous Eating Behaviors

Why is it that when you walk into a party the first thing that catches your attention is the one person with what you would call the "perfect" body? Glancing out of the corner of your eye, you turn green with envy. This person looks the way you've always wanted to look—thin, toned, and attractive. You'd die for a body like that. So, once again you vow to try just about anything to attain physical perfection, including taking extreme measures to lose weight and keep it off. And you may succeed, for a while, achieving the appearance you want. But what does it cost you? Maybe your health and well-being. And when you fail to reach physical perfection, you wind up feeling frustrated and bad about yourself once again.

---

*"At some point, you may stop and wonder how
the quest to lose weight became so all consuming."*

The drive to be thin can become an obsession when your thoughts continually focus on weight, size, body shape, food, calories, and fat grams. Notice how many times a day your mind drifts off to thoughts about appearance and food. You can put so much energy into these thoughts that your job and personal relationships begin to suffer. At some point, you may stop and wonder how the quest to lose weight became so all consuming.

Unhealthy eating patterns often develop quite innocently. You try a new diet and manage to lose some excess pounds. Your goal is to lose weight and feel good about yourself. You begin to believe that if you can attain physical perfection or something close to it, then everything in life will feel wonderful. And for a while it does. Friends and family members rave about how great you look, and your desire to become as thin as possible becomes stronger. But thin is never thin enough. You restrict your caloric intake even more with the hope of losing more weight. Yet, it's impossible to feel physically good when eating so little. So you overeat because you feel hungry and deprived. Overeating can then lead to more restrictive dieting, excessive exercise, purging, or taking substances to reduce hunger—diet pills, cocaine, crack, speed (also known as crystal), or ephedrine (an asthma medication). Because you can't stay on a diet forever, your weight yo-yos up or down depending on whether you're dieting or overeating. At that point, you're likely to develop a pattern of starving, bingeing, purging, or grazing.

These behaviors eventually become more than a method of weight control, however. They evolve into a complex coping mechanism that you use to deal with painful feelings and stressful life events. In these instances, food serves many purposes besides nourishing the body. As a matter of fact, you rarely consider food for its nutritional value, instead you eat it for its soothing effect and for distraction.

When you first lose weight, your self-esteem improves, and you're able to avoid uncomfortable emotions. As the behaviors become more entrenched and habitual, however, you begin to feel out of control. You start to believe you can't stop the behaviors even if you try, and you may be right. You feel stuck in a cycle that seems impossible to break. Any sense of self-worth you had gained now decreases as you struggle harder to maintain what you've achieved. You're overcome with self-loathing because engaging in these behaviors isn't working, your emotions are still painful and you can't maintain a permanent weight loss. Although you may really want to stop the unhealthy habits, you fear that giving up ingrained behaviors will lead to disaster—weight gain.

Striving for perfection can affect other areas of your life besides your appearance. In addition to wanting to look perfect, you may feel a constant inner push to "be the best" at work, school, and in relationships. Much of your energy is directed toward creating success and avoiding failure. But, for the most part, the successes seem short-lived and the failures are inevitable. You hope that success will create a constant sense of happiness, self-appreciation, and self-worth; it doesn't. Yet you persevere, hoping your actions will again result in success. You're not alone. This pattern of striving for perfection is universal among women and men who struggle with food issues.

People vary in terms of the seriousness of their unhealthy eating patterns. Many have mild problems with food and weight and so aren't distressed or concerned. Serious problems arise when someone develops an obsession with food and thinness, making it impossible to change eating behaviors that are considered abnormal. If you weren't concerned about your habits, you wouldn't be reading this workbook.

RECOGNIZING HARMFUL HABITS

There are four types of eating behaviors that become harmful and destructive—starving, bingeing, purging, and grazing. People striving to attain physical, emotional, and mental perfection often engage in one or more of these behaviors. In fact, you may find yourself falling into several of these categories.

Starving

Melody lost 45 pounds in five months. She now weighs just under 95 pounds, much too low a weight for her five-foot-six-inch height. She looks gaunt to others, but in her mirror she still sees an unattractive, overweight woman. So she continues to starve herself, hoping to achieve an unreachable perfection.

In the beginning, Melody dieted and lost weight. Over time, however, that weight loss took on a life of its own. Now, she feels controlled by the starvation but denies that it's a problem. If she admits she has a problem, she'll have to acknowledge her inability to stop starving herself and concede that she needs help. Instead, she claims she's not hungry, declaring that one orange, bagel, banana and nonfat yogurt a day are sufficient to keep her going. Meanwhile, she cooks for her boyfriend and watches him eat, but doesn't allow herself to eat any of that food.

Bouts of dizziness have begun to interfere with her ability to concentrate at work, which has her concerned. Plus it's taking more and more effort for her to look and act as if nothing's wrong. Melody even layers her clothing to make her look as if she weighs more than she actually does. The starvation is beginning to take a toll.

Dieting seems like the ideal solution to weight problems. TV, radio, magazines, and movies say it's true, equating thinness with happiness and success. However, dieting becomes starvation when the dieter restricts the caloric intake so extremely that weight loss occurs quickly. A starvation diet can mean eating as few as 500 calories a day. The minimum amount of calories consumed per day should be no fewer than 1,200. Cut below that, and the metabolic rate slows down to compensate for the lack of fuel needed to run the body. The body reacts by storing all incoming food in its reserves—the fat cells. The body will eat muscle before it eats fat, as a way to stay alive as long as possible. Ultimately, the body is trying to prevent premature death. For these reasons, starvation is a serious problem.

Starving causes a person to become intensely focused on food. It's not uncommon for people who are starving to talk about food, dream about food, prepare food for other people, watch cooking shows, and take cooking classes. So even though the body is deprived of food, the mind is obsessed with it.

Starving can become a coping mechanism for painful emotional experiences and stressful events. When your life feels out of control, the one thing you have ultimate control over is your body. So when you're faced with uncomfortable feelings or situations in which you believe you have little say, starving your body feels powerful, helping you right the balance of power and control. Over time, however, starving begins to make you feel out of control, yet stopping it seems impossible. Eating moderate amounts of food is incredibly frightening for a person caught up in the starvation cycle, so maintaining the starvation stance becomes easier than learning to eat again.

"Anorexics use one of two methods to maintain weight loss: they either restrict calories only, or they engage in bingeing and purging."

Constant starving over a period of time can develop into anorexia nervosa. You probably have anorexia if you have all of the following symptoms[1].

- Your body weight is less than 85 percent of what is considered normal for your age and height.

- You have an intense fear of gaining weight or becoming fat, even though you're actually underweight.

- You do not accurately perceive your weight, size, or shape (i.e., you "feel fat" even though you're actually emaciated).

- You're female and have missed three consecutive menstrual cycles.

Anorexics use one of two methods to maintain weight loss: they either restrict calories only, or they engage in *bingeing* and *purging*. Anorexics often use excessive and extreme amounts of exercise as their method of purging unwanted calories.

When a person continually deprives his or her body of food, the resulting weight loss can cause serious health problems and potentially irreversible damage. Physical complications associated with anorexia include damage to the heart and other vital organs, low blood pressure, slowed heartbeat, electrolyte imbalance (where sodium, potassium, and chloride are leached from the body causing cardiac arrhythmias, fatigue, muscle weakness, constipation, and depression), decreased metabolic rate, malnutrition, and abdominal pain, loss of muscle mass, hair loss, sensitivity to cold, fine body hair growth, dizziness, and impaired attention, retention, and concentration. Anorexics who engage in bingeing and purging have physical problems similar to bulimics.

Whether or not you fit the criteria for anorexia nervosa, starving is serious. It will never be the right solution. You must learn to eat food again, otherwise you'll literally waste away.

[1] American Psychiatric Association. *Diagnostic and Statistical Manual of Mental Disorders (4th Edition)*. Washington, D.C.: APA, 1994.

Bingeing

Bonnie has a problem and she knows it—she's a compulsive overeater. One moment she eats an entire box of donuts. Minutes later, she vows never to do that again. Yet the desire to binge on donuts, cookies, cake, or bread smothered in jam just "comes upon her." She feels angry and frustrated because she can't control herself. She almost believes there's a monster inside her making her behave this way.

Bonnie spends much of her time, energy, and money on junk food. She alternates between bingeing on food and scouring the latest women's magazines for the newest fad diet. She can stick to a diet for a few days or weeks, but eventually falls off because she feels hungry and deprived. Then she winds up gorging on all the things she couldn't eat while she was on the diet. What angers her most is that she weighs more now than ever before.

Her habits are also affecting her marriage. Bonnie refuses to leave the house if she "feels fat." So when she's dieting, she'll go out with her husband. When she's bingeing, she stays at home, holed up in their bedroom, leaving the house only to go to work or run necessary errands. Her husband feels crazed by this behavior. Bonnie knows this but doesn't know how to stop the binge/diet cycle.

Bingeing means eating large amounts of food in a short period of time. High-sugar, high-fat, and high-salt items are the snacks of choice because of their soothing, calming, and numbing qualities. The word bingeing implies more than just a behavior. Bingeing also means using food in a compulsive manner for reasons other than nourishing the body when it's hungry. It can seem like the best way to avoid unpleasant emotions stirred up by stressful experiences. Bingeing can take many forms. For some people, bingeing is eating large quantities between meals. For others, it's overeating during meals. And yet for others, it's eating more than they had originally planned at any one time. When the binge is over, however, the feelings are still there...plus the compulsive overeater has new feelings of self-disgust and self-loathing with which to cope. Because the behavior is so embarrassing and brings such shame, compulsive overeaters generally eat alone and in secret, unless they find a binge buddy (another person to binge with).

Compulsive overeaters feel compelled to eat for a variety of reasons. Do any of these sound familiar? You eat:

- Out of habit

- As a temporary escape from strong emotions or stressful situations

- After depriving yourself of food for some time

- Because once you begin a meal you're unable to stop eating

Notice how many times a day food and eating enter your mind. Do you spend hours thinking about and planning binges? Bingeing can become so distracting that it affects work projects and relationships, making them seem less important than bingeing.

Compulsive overeaters frequently alternate between bingeing and dieting. Yet the diets never lead to permanent weight loss. Those who binge usually gain more weight after coming off a diet than before they started it. After so many failed attempts to permanently lose weight, the dieter begins to experience self-blame and to feel angry and disgusted, a weak-willed failure. In reality, bingeing is often an automatic reaction to restrictive diets that leave the body feeling hungry. The body needs more food than most diets allow for. In fact, up to 95 percent of dieters fail to keep the weight off. And few, if any, diets have proven effective for permanent weight loss, meaning the weight stays off two or more years and the person never has to diet again. That's why most dieters have attempted so many different kinds of diet plans.

> *"Often, bingers spend more money*
> *on food than on anything else."*

People try all sorts of programs to lose weight. Some sign up with diet businesses that promote weight loss and sell special food products. Then there are diet shakes, diet books, diet pills, nutritional formulas and supplements, and extreme exercise regimens that claim to enhance weight loss. Some desperate people even try taking drugs like syrup of ipecac to induce vomiting, or ephedrine, cocaine, crack, or speed to reduce hunger pangs. These rarely create any permanent weight loss, nor do they help change unhealthy eating patterns into healthy ones. They're hardly solutions you can use for the rest of your life.

Continued bingeing behavior can be expensive. Often, bingers spend more money on food than on anything else. If you're a binger, stop and calculate how much money you spend on bingeing, diet programs, and diet books. You'll be surprised at how much all this is costing you. Yet you feel driven and out of control, as if the overeating is controlling you, you're no longer controlling it. A quick, numbing solution to life's problems has become a catalyst for creating future problems.

Compulsive overeating has recently been given the diagnostic label "binge eating disorder."[2] The criteria for this disorder include:

- Recurrent episodes of binge eating where large amounts of food are eaten in a discrete period of time (within a two-hour period)

- A sense of lack of control over eating during the episode

- Feeling distress about binge eating

[2] American Psychiatric Association. *Diagnostic and Statistical Manual of Mental Disorders (4th Edition)*. Washington, D.C.: APA, 1994.

- Any three of the following:

  * Eating more rapidly than normal

  * Eating until uncomfortably full

  * Eating large amounts of food when not physically hungry

  * Eating alone because you're embarrassed by how much you eat

  * Feeling disgusted, depressed, or guilty after binge eating

Compulsive overeating can lead to weight gain and obesity. Physical complications associated with long-term weight problems include diabetes, hypertension, circulatory problems, degenerative joint disease, cardiovascular disease, and hormonal imbalances. Yet, this is often not enough to prevent bingeing. What you do know is that bingeing doesn't work and neither does dieting. When you stop bingeing and start eating normally, you'll lose pounds slowly and ultimately reach a healthy weight.

Purging

Sandy binges on large amounts of food and then vomits to get the food out of her body. Sometimes she uses laxatives or diuretics to force the food through her system more quickly. She started bingeing and purging once or twice a month about two years ago when she felt stressed out. Now she does it every day, sometimes as much as four times a day. She knows the location of all the convenience stores for her binge food buying and has figured out where she can purge on her college campus. She makes sure she alternates where she shops and which bathrooms she visits. Sandy feels out of control and stuck. The thought of giving up the bingeing and purging scares her. She believes she'll gain weight if she eats regularly and keeps the food down. You'd never suspect that Sandy has a problem by the way she looks. Most people would consider her thin and attractive, yet Sandy doesn't see herself that way.

Purging is a behavior used to rid the body of unwanted food and calories after eating. It can also create a sense of being purified or cleansed. You've alleviated the guilt of overeating, expelled the food, and have a fresh opportunity to start anew. Purging can take on many forms including self-induced vomiting; misuse of laxatives, diuretics, enemas, or other medications; fasting; or excessive exercise. There are a number of ways in which people discover how to purge. Some learn by accident, others by trial and error, or when a friend, coworker, or magazine article discusses how to do it. Purging seems like the ultimate solution; you can eat whatever you want and not gain weight. However, research has shown that about 1,200 calories are retained in the body regardless of how much food was consumed during a binge (unless the binge was less than 1,200 calories) or how many efforts were made to purge the food. The reason for this is the stomach and bowel seem to absorb and process food at a fixed rate, no matter what is done to try and get rid of it.

While purging seems to work in the beginning, over time it takes on a life of its own, compelling you to purge every time you eat or overeat. When the behavior gets out of control, though, it can be frightening, becoming a habit that seems impossible to break.

If you are bingeing and purging, you may have bulimia nervosa, a disorder for which the symptoms include:[3]

- Recurrent episodes of binge eating

- Feeling a lack of control over eating during the binges

- Engaging in recurrent compensatory behaviors (purging) to prevent weight gain from bingeing

- Engaging in bingeing and purging at least twice a week for three months

- Being unduly influenced by body shape and weight when evaluating yourself

Some anorexics binge and purge to maintain extreme weight loss. Sometimes they don't eat enough food to classify it as a binge, yet they purge anyway.

Purging can create physical complications that include damage to the heart, kidneys, reproductive system, intestinal tract, esophagus, teeth, and mouth. Vomiting and laxatives or diuretic abuse can cause malnutrition and dehydration. Purging also creates an electrolyte imbalance because it drains water, sodium, potassium, and chloride from the body. This can lead to cardiac arrhythmias, constipation, fatigue, muscle weakness, and depression. Mental capabilities such as concentration, attention, and retention are affected as well. Because purging is dangerous, it must be stopped before it leads to irreparable physical problems.

Grazing

Matt is a grazer—which means he's eating something pretty much all the time. Because of this, he weighs 30 pounds more than is healthy for him. Often, Matt goes for weeks without sitting down to a regular meal unless he goes out to dinner with friends. He finds himself thinking about food constantly. Right after he finishes eating, he's planning what he is going to buy and eat next. He even fantasizes about food and what it's going to taste like. A big bag of candy sits nearby in his drawer at work and he picks at it all day long. He feels distracted at work and less productive than he once was. His job doesn't seem fun compared to eating. He knows something isn't quite right in his life but doesn't know what to do about it.

---

[3] American Psychiatric Association. *Diagnostic and Statistical Manual of Mental Disorders (4th Edition).* Washington, D.C.: APA, 1994.

People who graze eat from morning to evening without having designated meal times. The whole day is one long snacking event. Grazers usually choose foods that are easily accessible and take little or no preparation. For them, it seems impossible to fix a meal, sit at the table, enjoy the meal, and stop when finished. When they do sit down to a meal, they find they can't stop eating, and they go on to graze for the rest of the day or evening.

Grazers often eat unhealthy quantities of food and make poor food choices. Their top choices are usually quick, easy, and high in sugar, fat, or salt. You rarely find fruits, vegetables, and grains on their plate. This behavior, not surprisingly, often results in a weight gain, since they consume many more calories than needed. It would be hard for them to calculate how many calories were eaten because they snack throughout the day. This constant eating doesn't allow the body to register messages about satiation, so they never know whether they're hungry or full.

"The longer you've engaged in unhealthy patterns,
the more pronounced your symptoms are likely to be."

Like other unhealthy eating styles, grazing becomes distressing when it begins to feel out of control, when eating regular meals seems impossible, when dieting hasn't worked, and when food is used to numb unpleasant emotions. Grazing is different than choosing to eat four to six smaller meals a day without feeling out of control or using food to cope with painful life events. People may decide to eat more than three meals a day for a variety of reasons: it keeps their blood/sugar level constant, they have more energy, their physician recommends it, or it fits into their busy lifestyle. Because both grazing and eating meals are learned behaviors, grazers can learn to eat three meals a day (with snacks, if necessary) just as they've learned to graze.

Assignment: Assess which of the four types of harmful eating behaviors—starving, bingeing, purging, or grazing—you engage in and their severity. Spend time thinking about your struggle with food, weight, and body-image, and about how this has adversely affected your life. Understanding your behaviors will help you see that the pursuit of thinness has developed into a coping mechanism for life's ups and downs.

The next chapter provides a list of physical as well as emotional and mental symptoms associated with unhealthy eating behaviors and the resulting weight problems. The longer you've engaged in these patterns, the more pronounced your symptoms are likely to be. Most people who struggle with food, weight, and body image share similar physical, emotional, and mental symptoms. To begin healing, you must identify your individual symptoms.

1 - 4

The Body Factor:
Determining Your Physical Symptoms

The body is amazingly resilient. It can tolerate all kinds of neglect…for a while. That's why it's hard to believe your eating habits are actually harming your health. In fact, many physical symptoms take time to develop. However, eventually the body begins to feel the effects of starving, bingeing, purging, or grazing. Physical symptoms that used to come and go now take more time to heal. And some symptoms don't seem to go away at all. This is a clear sign that the behaviors are beginning to take their toll. Deciding to change unhealthy eating patterns means first assessing what effects the harmful behaviors have had on your body. You may be noticing a number of symptoms and not know what they're related to or which behaviors have caused them. There may be other symptoms

---

"Many symptoms will go away once your eating becomes regular and moderate, and when you stop starving or purging."

---

for which you see a direct connection to your eating behaviors. Regular medical checkups can help you to understand any physical problems you're experiencing. But be honest with the physician about your current eating habits. You may even want to see a specialist who knows what to look for regarding health and weight problems brought on by harmful eating patterns. Many symptoms will go away once your eating becomes regular and moderate, and when you stop starving or purging.

Assignment: Fill out the following checklist to determine which symptoms, if any, you're experiencing. Physical symptoms are your body's way of telling you how your eating habits are affecting you. After you complete the exercises in this workbook, fill out the checklist again, and use this as a measure to assess how many of your symptoms have decreased or gone away completely.

Rate the physical symptoms below by how often you experience them, using the five-point scale:

SCALE

Never	Rarely	Sometimes	Much of the Time	Most of the Time	All of the Time
0	1	2	3	4	5

	Times Symptoms Experienced (0-5) Now	Times Symptoms Experienced (0-5) After Using Workbook

Symptoms Related to Weight:

Weight fluctuates +/− 10 pounds	_____	_____
Weigh 20% above recommended weight	_____	_____
Weigh 15% below recommended weight	_____	_____
Despite eating less food, you can't lose weight	_____	_____
Eat very few calories and still gain weight	_____	_____
Subtotal	_____	_____

Symptoms Related to the Head and Throat:

Headaches	_____	_____
Dizziness	_____	_____
Poor concentration, attention, and retention	_____	_____
Hair loss	_____	_____
Constant thirst	_____	_____
Blisters in throat (due to vomiting)	_____	_____
Eroding teeth enamel (vomiting)	_____	_____
Gum disease (vomiting)	_____	_____
Swollen salivary glands	_____	_____
Subtotal	_____	_____

Symptoms Related to the Body and Muscles:

Fatigue or lethargy	_____	_____
Muscle weakness	_____	_____

Muscle cramps	_____	_____
Achy joints	_____	_____
Water retention (e.g., swollen face, hands, ankles, feet)	_____	_____
Sensitivity to the cold	_____	_____
Fine body hair growth	_____	_____
Brittle fingernails	_____	_____
Scaly skin	_____	_____
Subtotal	======	======

Symptoms Related to the Digestive Tract:

Difficulty keeping food down	_____	_____
Difficulty swallowing	_____	_____
Digestive problems	_____	_____
Stomach cramping	_____	_____
Constipation	_____	_____
Diarrhea	_____	_____
Nausea	_____	_____
Subtotal	======	======

Symptoms Related to the Heart, Lungs, Kidneys, and Pancreas:

Heart palpitations	_____	_____
Slowed pulse rate	_____	_____
High blood pressure	_____	_____
Heart disease	_____	_____
Electrolyte imbalance	_____	_____
Difficulty with breathing	_____	_____
Circulatory problems	_____	_____
Kidney problems	_____	_____
Diabetes	_____	_____
Subtotal	======	======

Symptoms Related to the Female Reproductive System:

Complete loss of menstruation	_____	_____
Periodic loss of menstruation	_____	_____
Subtotal	======	======

Overall Total Score	======	======

Scoring: Add up all the subtotals for each group of symptoms, then compute your score. The total score indicates the severity of physical symptoms.

1.	Mild	=	1 – 41
2.	Moderate	=	42 – 82
3.	Serious	=	83 – 123
4.	Severe	=	124 – 164
5.	Critical	=	165 – 205

Pay particular attention to the symptoms for which you score 4 or 5. These individual scores may indicate physical symptoms that need immediate attention.

The best way to understand your particular symptomatology is to calculate the total score before you do the exercises in the workbook and then again after you finish the workbook. Compare the individual items as well as the total score for each testing to see which physical symptoms have decreased and which ones no longer exist.

Symptoms Needing *Immediate* Attention

If you answer YES to any of the following questions, consult your physician immediately.

1. Are you dizzy or fainting? _____
2. Are you fatigued much of the time? _____
3. Do you have ongoing heart palpitations? _____
4. Are you having difficulty keeping food down? _____
5. Do you have severe stomach pains or cramps? _____
6. Do you have severe constipation? _____
7. Do you have continual diarrhea? _____
8. Do you see blood when you vomit? _____
9. Do you have bloody bowel movements? _____
10. Do you have chronic lower back or kidney pain? _____
11. Do you have severe throat pain? _____
12. Do you have chronic and extreme chest pain? _____
13. Do you have difficulty breathing? _____
14. Are your teeth extremely sensitive to heat or cold? _____
15. Are you losing your hair? _____

Note: The checklist of physical symptoms is not intended to be used as a diagnostic measurement, but as an opportunity for self-awareness. You can use this list to examine the physical symptoms you're currently experiencing. This can help you gain more understanding and create change.

1 - 5

Your Heart and Head:
Measuring Your Emotional and Mental Symptoms

Recognizing and dealing with painful emotions and negative thinking is never easy or comfortable. Consequently, many people use food—eating too much or too little—as a way of coping with feelings and thoughts they believe they shouldn't have or that overwhelm them. Bingeing, purging, grazing, or starving become the standard way to handle life's ups and downs.

"You can change your beliefs and attitudes,
and process and release your emotions."

Your feelings are fueled by negative beliefs and attitudes you hold about yourself, other people, and the world in general. To make sense of your feelings, and to support and reinforce those beliefs, you begin to think in a certain predictable pattern. Many feelings often seem too complex and all-consuming to handle or even examine, and there seems to be no escape from this negative or distorted thinking.

Once you recognize how your beliefs lead to emotional reactions and negative thinking, then you can learn to deal with both your feelings and your thoughts. You can change your beliefs and attitudes, and process and release your emotions. Some painful feelings and negative thoughts will decrease in intensity once you begin to regulate your eating. This is because you're no longer engaging in behaviors that are distressing and lead to self-hatred. Other feelings will seem stronger and more pressing because they're not being masked by the effects of food.

Assignment: Complete the following checklist to determine which emotional and mental symptoms you're currently experiencing. Become aware of what thoughts and feelings are fueling your food issues. Return to this checklist after you have completed the workbook and compare the two results to measure how many symptoms have diminished or disappeared completely.

Rate how often you experience the following emotional and mental symptoms, using the five-point scale:

SCALE

Never	Rarely	Sometimes	Much of the Time	Most of the Time	All of the Time
0	1	2	3	4	5

	Times Symptoms Experienced (0-5) Now	Times Symptoms Experienced (0-5) After Using Workbook

Symptoms Related to Depression:

Feel down or blue	_____	_____
Feel "blah"	_____	_____
Feel sad	_____	_____
Cry more than usual	_____	_____
Feel like the weight of the world is on your shoulders	_____	_____
Get less satisfaction from things than in the past	_____	_____
Difficulty with concentration	_____	_____
Difficulty with making decisions	_____	_____
Less motivated than usual	_____	_____
Feel like a failure	_____	_____
Feel moody or irritated	_____	_____
Feel discouraged about the future	_____	_____
Sleep too much or too little	_____	_____
Diminished interest in sex	_____	_____
Feel hopeless at times	_____	_____
Subtotal	_____	_____

Symptoms Related to Anxiety:

Tightness in your chest	_____	_____
A sinking feeling	_____	_____
A fear of dying	_____	_____
A fear of going crazy	_____	_____

Physiological Symptoms:

Shortness of breath   _____   _____

Heart palpitations   _____   _____

Chest pain   _____   _____

Choking   _____   _____

Sweating   _____   _____

Dry mouth   _____   _____

Skin flushes   _____   _____

Muscle tension   _____   _____

Trembling   _____   _____

Restlessness   _____   _____

Subtotal   =======   =======

Symptoms Related to Low Self-Esteem:

Highly self-critical   _____   _____

Unrealistic expectations of yourself   _____   _____

Overly sensitive to criticism from others   _____   _____

Feel worthless   _____   _____

Feel powerless   _____   _____

Feel helpless   _____   _____

Subtotal   =======   =======

Symptoms Related to Perfectionism:

Want to control all situations   _____   _____

Want to control others   _____   _____

Need to be perfect at everything   _____   _____

Appearance needs to be perfect   _____   _____

Cannot make mistakes   _____   _____

Subtotal   =======   =======

Symptoms Related to Interpersonal Relationships:

Need constant approval   _____   _____

Have difficulty being assertive   _____   _____

Have difficulty saying "no"   _____   _____

Want to continually please others   _____   _____

Take care of other's needs before your own   _____   _____

Isolate yourself from others   _____   _____

Described by others as moody or irritable   _____   _____

Subtotal   =======   =======

Symptoms Related to Body Image:

You "feel fat"   _____   _____
Are preoccupied with your weight   _____   _____
Critical or jealous of other people's weight or appearance   _____   _____
See yourself as heavier than you actually are   _____   _____
Wear baggy or layered clothing to hide weight loss _____   _____
Subtotal   _____   _____

Symptoms Related to Obsessive Thoughts and Compulsive Behaviors:

Have obsessive thoughts you cannot stop   _____   _____
Have compulsive behaviors you cannot stop   _____   _____
Exercise beyond what is considered moderate   _____   _____
Fix your hair, makeup or clothing throughout the day _____   _____
Neat to the point of letting the slightest dirt or
    disorganization bother you   _____   _____
  Are impulsive in a number of areas:
  Impulse buying   _____   _____
  Shoplifting   _____   _____
  Sexually promiscuous   _____   _____
  Use drugs or alcohol like you use food   _____   _____
Subtotal   _____   _____

Symptoms Related to Eating Behaviors:

Secretive about what and when you eat   _____   _____
Afraid of food   _____   _____
Tense at meals   _____   _____
Avoid certain foods   _____   _____
Avoid eating with others   _____   _____
Restrict food in public and binge in private   _____   _____
Fear you cannot stop eating once you start   _____   _____
  Engage in eating rituals:
  Count number of times food is chewed   _____   _____
  Count bites   _____   _____
  Make food last as long as possible   _____   _____
  Eat so quickly that you don't taste the food _____   _____
  Eat only one food at a time   _____   _____
  Binge on "junk food," diet on "healthy food" _____   _____
  Chew food and spit it out instead of swallowing _____   _____
  Separate foods on the plate into distinct piles
      eating only one pile at a time _____   _____

Wait until evening to eat your first meal   _____   _____
     Eat "forbidden" foods in secret   _____   _____
Subtotal   ======   ======

Overall Total Score   ======   ======

Scoring: Add up all the numbers given for each question and compute a total score. The score indicates the severity of emotional and mental symptoms.

1.	Mild	=	1 – 78
2.	Moderate	=	79 – 156
3.	Serious	=	157 – 234
4.	Severe	=	235 – 312
5.	Critical	=	313 – 390

Pay particular attention to the questions for which you score a 4 or 5. These individual scores may indicate emotional and mental symptoms that need immediate attention.

To best understand your particular symptoms, calculate the total score before you do the exercises in the workbook and then again after you finish the workbook. Compare the scores for each individual item as well as the total scores to see which symptoms have decreased and which ones no longer exist.

Symptoms Needing *Immediate* Attention

If you answer YES to any of the questions below, consult a mental health practitioner immediately.

1. Are you experiencing severe depression?   _____
2. Are you having panic attacks?   _____
3. Are you having anxiety attacks?   _____
4. Are you experiencing extreme obsessive thoughts?   _____
5. Are you experiencing extreme compulsive behavior?   _____
6. Are you having suicidal thoughts or making suicide attempts?   _____

Note: The checklist of emotional and mental symptoms above is not intended to be used as a diagnostic measurement, but rather as an opportunity for self-awareness. You can use this list to examine the symptoms you're currently experiencing. From this information, you can gain more understanding to help you make necessary changes.

WHERE YOU ARE NOW

By the end of **Part One: Unhealthy Eating Behaviors,** you'll have a clear idea of the types of harmful food habits you engage in and the effect they're having on your body and mind. If you desire, go back to the areas you want to explore more fully. Check (✓) the areas you've completed.

_____ You've assessed the signs that relate to your harmful eating behaviors and how to become healthier physically, emotionally, mentally, and spiritually.

_____ You've set up a realistic schedule for using this workbook that will promote success.

_____ You've identified your own unique set of unhealthy eating behaviors and the severity with which you experience them.

_____ You've determined your physical symptoms and know what your body is currently experiencing because of your eating patterns.

_____ You've measured your emotional and mental symptoms and understand what thoughts and feelings fuel your food abuse.

With all the information you now have about your particular eating behaviors, you're ready to move on to **Part Two: Healing the Physical Self.**

PART TWO:
HEALING
THE
PHYSICAL
SELF

2 - 1

Why Do I Keep Doing This?: Breaking the Food Addiction Cycle

Peg hurries into the grocery store with one thing on her mind—food! She's not thinking about the weekly shopping for her family though; she's on a mission to find something rich and decadent to eat. At the moment, Peg has tunnel vision. She left any thought of, "Why am I doing this?" outside the store. Carefully scanning the aisles for the perfect treat, she cruises past the pastry counter, up the cookie aisle, down by the candy bins, and on to the freezer section. Aha! A tube of raw cookie dough. Just what she saw advertised on TV last night. Peg figures she can eat this in the car while driving home, then have rocky road ice cream while finishing up the work she brought from the office. Tonight's the perfect night for a binge because her son and husband are at a baseball game. They'll never know that she had ice cream for dinner.

Only briefly does Peg consider the consequences of a binge. Before pushing it out of her mind, she grabs a pack of diet pills and promises herself she will take them in the morning. Serious regrets set in only after she's finished stuffing down the cookie dough and ice cream. "Why do I keep doing this?" she thinks, angry with herself once again. She vows never, ever to binge again...the same promise she made to herself yesterday and the day before.

"Unhealthy eating patterns can be as addictive as alcohol, drugs, gambling, and impulse shopping."

Peg is not alone. Many people struggle with the addictive nature of food and unhealthy eating patterns, which can be as addictive as alcohol, drugs, gambling, and impulse shopping. Much like other addictions, harmful eating behaviors are infrequent in the beginning. You may think a quick fad diet to lose weight, an occasional binge just to indulge, or purging here and there to prevent weight gain are all pretty innocent. In the beginning they might be. But months or years later, the behaviors will have become all-consuming, and you'll feel powerless to change them.

The addictive process actually occurs rather slowly and insidiously, growing until it reaches a point where food and the behaviors surrounding the food begin to take over. When you make decisions that damage your health, personal relationships, and job, the behavior (starving, bingeing, or purging) is controlling you, you're not controlling it.

> *"Research has shown that carbohydrates release the brain chemical serotonin, which is believed to reduce feelings of anxiety and frustration."*

For many, bingeing or grazing on food can be soothing and distracting, helping the eater cope with uncomfortable emotions and stressful experiences. Carbohydrates have a calming effect on the body, consequently the snack foods that people generally choose for bingeing or grazing are high in carbohydrates (and often high in fat): items like donuts, cookies, cakes, candy, chips, breads, pastas, and potatoes. Simple carbohydrates are found in sugar, honey, syrups, and molasses. Complex carbohydrates are found in grains, beans, vegetables, and fruits. Research has shown that carbohydrates release the brain chemical serotonin, which is believed to reduce feelings of anxiety and frustration. Chocolate, which is made up of sugars and fat, contains phenylethylamine, which is also known to decrease depression and anxiety.

Purging or starving may seem like the perfect solution once you've put on too many pounds or feel panicked about gaining weight. And for those who only starve themselves and have never binged, there is a great sense of power in being able to maintain a starvation stance. However, what started out as feeling good begins to spiral out of control. When other areas of your life feel unmanageable and beyond your control, the one thing you have ultimate control over is your body. You have the final say as to what you do to your body, deciding how much it's fed and how much it weighs, at least in the beginning stages. As time goes on, it becomes harder to manipulate either weight or food intake.

Harmful eating patterns become habitual and cyclical. The cycle begins with a stressful event that triggers unpleasant feelings (e.g., anger, guilt, hurt, frustration, sadness, self-loathing). This leads to a negative thought or interpretation about yourself and sometimes the stressful event. So you turn to ineffective coping behaviors such as bingeing, purging, starving, or grazing to deal with your feelings and thoughts. This creates more painful feelings and more negative thoughts because you're ashamed and unhappy about your eating patterns. The cycle gets replayed over and over again. The diagram below illustrates the process.

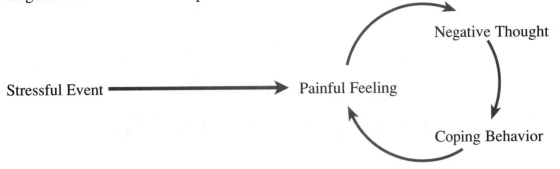

Stressful Event ⟶ Painful Feeling → Negative Thought → Coping Behavior →

Break one link in the chain of events and the cycle is thrown off. Then you can make adjustments in other parts of the cycle. This creates an opportunity to decrease and eventually stop the behavior. For example, if you binge and purge, and you stop bingeing, then the need for purging is eliminated. By eliminating both of these behaviors, you reduce the negative feelings that get stirred up by the bingeing and purging. Breaking the cycle provides an opportunity for you to find other, healthier ways of dealing with the original stressful event, the emotions that arise, and the accompanying negative thoughts.

"One of the most important areas for you to address is how you think about and approach food on a daily basis."

Be warned. This isn't an easy task. It takes time and energy to make these changes. But you *can* do it. This workbook will give you a variety of techniques and strategies to help you learn to break the vicious cycle of unhealthy eating patterns and the weight problems that result from them.

One of the most important areas for you to address is how you think about and approach food on a daily basis. This chapter will help you understand food behaviors, change your eating habits, and find new ways of coping with life's unavoidable pressures.

Assignment: Explore why you've become caught up in the cycle of turning to, denying yourself, or purging food to cope with stressful events or unpleasant emotions. Think about one or two changes you can make to break the cycle.

2 - 2

Diets Make You Fatter:
Eat Your Way to a Healthy Weight

Diets make you fatter! Dieting has never been an effective way to control weight because depriving your body of food does two things that work against you. First, low-calorie dieting creates a continual feeling of hunger that leads to obsessive thoughts of food.

"In our society, overeating is interpreted as a lack of willpower. In reality, bingeing is the body's way of making sure you get enough food after you've stopped restrictive dieting."

When you stop dieting, your eating often goes out of control. You binge on the "forbidden" foods you denied yourself while dieting.

In our society, overeating is interpreted as a lack of willpower. In reality, bingeing is the body's way of making sure you get enough food after you've stopped restrictive dieting. Your body cannot tell the difference between intentional dieting and a famine. All it knows is it's not getting enough food, and to make sure it doesn't starve to death, the body will overcompensate for the times when it was deprived.

Diet programs are not geared toward permanent weight loss. Few, if any, diets have proven effective for long-term weight loss (two years or more). This is because diets don't teach healthy eating patterns that you can follow for the rest of your life without ever having to diet again. Nor do they teach you how to shop for and prepare food, or how to eat anything you want within moderation and still lose weight permanently. They teach deprivation, which pushes you to binge on the foods you couldn't have while dieting. That's why it's so easy to return to the old, familiar eating behaviors and why you then have to go back to dieting.

The second reason diets don't work is that eating less food actually makes it harder to lose weight. Dieting fights against the body's weight-regulating mechanism located in the brain. This control center chooses a "setpoint" weight based on the amount of body fat it considers ideal for your needs. When you diet restrictively, the mechanism will work to keep weight on, believing it needs that weight to survive. So if you eat less food, your body slows down its metabolic rate to compensate for the fewer calories consumed. When you eat less, you burn fewer calories. Conversely, if you eat more, your metabolism will burn more. For instance, a 500-calorie-a-day diet lowers the metabolic rate 15 to 20 percent below normal. So the longer you diet, the harder it is to lose weight and the easier it is to gain weight.

"Muscle burns calories. That's why exercise is recommended as a healthy form of weight control—it increases muscle mass."

The body also stores any incoming fat in fat cells to make sure there's a reserve for the next time food is restricted. While on a diet, your body begins trying to store fat. When you come off a diet and eat more food, you'll actually store more fat. Your fat cells help you survive restrictive diets by becoming larger, stronger, and more resistant.

Muscle burns calories. That's why exercise is recommended as a healthy form of weight control—it increases muscle mass. When you diet, your body wants to reduce the amount of muscle mass you have in order to slow down your metabolism and conserve energy. Therefore your metabolism is slower because you have less muscle. You can actually eat fewer calories than before and still gain weight. This problem gets worse with every new diet you undertake—storing more fat, losing muscle mass, and decreasing your metabolic rate. Dieting fights the body's weight-regulating system and, thus, is bound to fail.

When you alternate dieting or starving with bingeing, grazing, or purging, your metabolism doesn't know when your body is going to receive and retain food, so it slows down to prevent death. Therefore, restricting your caloric intake keeps your body weight higher than if you weren't dieting at all. You can weigh more after a bout of dieting than you weighed before you started the diet. Switching back and forth between restrictive dieting and eating high-fat foods, in addition to living a sedentary lifestyle, has led more people to becoming overweight in this country than ever before.

So what does work? Regular and moderate eating and exercise will increase your metabolic rate. The more foods you eat, the more calories you'll burn (unless the majority of the calories come from fat or you're not eating moderate amounts). The key is to eat a variety of foods, with the majority of calories (50–65 percent) from complex carbohydrates (grains, beans, fruits, and vegetables), 15–20 percent from protein, and about 20–30 percent of calories from fat. There has been a bias against eating carbohydrates in the past, based on the false belief that they make you gain weight. But it's either the fat you add to high-carbohydrate foods or eating too much of them that makes them fattening. In fact, they are the foods that fuel your body. You can actually eat anything you want, within reason—meaning that portion sizes are moderate (one to two servings), and you don't eat high-fat or high-sugar food all the time. High-fat or high-sugar foods can add to weight gain, especially if you binge on large amounts. When you want to have them, include them in reasonable portions within a meal, balancing them with healthy foods. The healthiest kind of foods are low in fats, salts, sugar, chemicals, and additives, and high in fiber and complex carbohydrates. So choose foods that are closest to their natural, preprocessed form—fresh fruits, vegetables, grains, and beans.

Eating regularly, usually three meals a day (with snacks, if needed), and eating when you're hungry and stopping when you're full helps with weight regulation. Your body knows when it needs to eat and it will tell you. You just need to begin listening to the messages. When you respond to hunger, you will feed your body the right amount of food at that time. Your metabolism burns those calories instead of storing them. If you eat the same amount of calories in one meal a day, you'll gain weight. Your body will store all the calories it didn't utilize in your fat cells. Then, after a number of hours, your body becomes hungry and waits to be fed. When it doesn't receive food, your metabolic rate slows down in anticipation of being starved. Both factors lead to weight gain.

"If you ate 100 fewer calories a day, you would lose ten pounds in a year."

With this formula of eating in moderation and with regularity, you can maintain a healthy weight or you can lose weight. To lose weight, you should never reduce caloric intake to the point of feeling deprived. That means you don't drop below 1,200 calories a day. Alter the kinds of foods you eat. Reduce the calories you get from fat to 20 percent or less a day. Increase the amounts of fruits, vegetables, and grains that you eat, making sure they're prepared in a healthful manner. Also, decrease the amount of high-sugar and high-salt items and choose moderate portion sizes. When you want dessert, eat it with your meal in a moderate amount (one serving size) instead of eventually bingeing on it because you feel deprived.

If you ate 100 fewer calories a day, you would lose ten pounds in a year. Not only is the weight loss more likely to be permanent, it's also quite effortless—you simply eat one less food item a day. For example, if you eat three 100-calorie cookies a day for your afternoon snack, have two cookies a day instead. The basic keys to successful weight loss are eating meals regularly, eating moderate amounts, choosing healthy foods, reducing fat intake, and eating foods you really desire. You will never have to diet, count calories, or estimate fat grams again. And you can eat this way for the rest of your life.

> *"Your body is very wise. It knows*
> *what it needs to weigh to be fit."*

Exercise is also a key ingredient for weight maintenance and weight loss. When you exercise in moderation, your setpoint will eventually readjust downward. This means that, over time, your body will want to weigh less without you having to impose rigid or harmful behaviors on it. Your body fat will decrease because your body doesn't need it. It's as if your body is telling the fat cells to get smaller and stay that way. This may sound paradoxical, perhaps even frightening, to eat and exercise regularly and moderately, and give up dieting. Yet it works. Initially, you might gain some weight, until your metabolism begins working efficiently. Once your metabolism is working at its optimum level, however, the pounds will come off slowly and your weight will stabilize.

Your body is very wise. It knows what it needs to weigh to be fit. This means allowing your body to decide what weight is naturally best for you. Trusting your body to pick the right weight can be difficult when you've been manipulating your weight for so long. When you treat your body well, it will respond by feeling better and weighing a healthy weight. This means that if you're overweight and you focus on changing your eating and exercise habits, the by-product will be eventual, permanent weight loss. When weight loss is the main focus, versus changing eating and exercise behaviors, it's easier to become obsessed with your weight. By paying attention to food and exercise, and deemphasizing weight loss, the obsession decreases, yet weight loss still occurs. Your body will pick a weight that's healthy, although it may not match the number or size in your head. That weight may take extreme measures to maintain, and your body may need to weigh more to stay healthy long term. Allow your body to be healthier by weighing what you need to weigh to function optimally.

Assignment: To see how dieting has failed you, fill out the *List Your Diets* chart. Be honest with yourself in assessing each diet's success and you'll begin to see a pattern of disappointments—either your weight stayed the same or you gained more weight than before you started the diet.

LIST YOUR DIETS

Make a list of the diets you have tried, when you tried each one, how much weight you lost, the length of time the weight stayed off, and how much weight you gained back.

DIET	WHEN	POUNDS LOST	TIME KEPT OFF	WEIGHT REGAINED

2 - 3

Three Meals a Day Keep the Weight Away: Make Time and Space to Eat

You've heard it before. Eat three scheduled meals a day. Yet this can seem unrealistic and even impossible to achieve, especially today when many of us lead such hectic lives.

"You consume many more calories during bingeing or grazing than you do when you eat three balanced meals."

The thought of trying to regulate your eating patterns or eat the amount of food generally advised by health practitioners who promote three meals a day seems difficult at best. Most people fear they'll gain weight or they won't be able to modify their habits. However, you consume many more calories during bingeing or grazing than you do when you eat three balanced meals.

Whether you're currently bingeing, starving, or grazing, it's important to work toward developing a consistent eating pattern. You can't diet for the rest of your life, but you can eat normally (whatever is normal for you). Do this, and your weight will stop yo-yoing and so will the weight gain. Your weight will actually stabilize and eventually decrease (unless you're anorexic, then weight gain is your goal).

Meal Planning

Meal planning implies deciding what you're going to eat beforehand, whether it's for the whole week, the next day, or an upcoming meal. What you want to avoid is impulse eating—choosing unhealthy foods because they taste good when you're famished. Impulse eating makes it more likely you'll eat haphazardly, not having any consistent pattern throughout the day, or from one day to the next. Planning does not necessarily mean making elaborate meals, although it can. You can decide a day or even an hour before you eat what you're hungry for and where you're going to get it.

The first step in developing a consistent eating pattern is to plan meals. Do this by grouping foods into separate meal times. Many people skip breakfast because they believe it sets them off—making them eat uncontrollably all day. Eating uncontrollably isn't caused by physiological cravings, unless you've deprived yourself of food for long periods of time. All other uncontrolled eating is due to psychological factors. Your body knows when it's full, although you may still want to eat for emotional reasons or out of habit. You need to eat breakfast so that your body will have something to run on. You haven't eaten since the night before, about twelve hours, and your body needs to be fed. You also need to eat lunch and dinner, with snacks in between if you get hungry. You'll feel much more "in control" of your eating if you eat planned meals and make healthier food choices. You'll also feel better physically. It's the bingeing and grazing that lead you to feel out of control.

In the beginning, portion size and moderation are less important than creating three separate meals. You want to create a habit of eating three meals a day, eating enough food at each meal so you feel satisfied, but not overeating to the point of feeling stuffed. Your goal is to make it so automatic to eat a meal that you do it without having to think about it or get stressed out over it, much like brushing your teeth.

Once you've developed a habit of eating three meals, then work on portion size and food choices. If you already eat three meals a day, begin now to focus on portion sizes and types of foods. Some people find it too difficult to plan three meals and they do better just regulating one meal, then adding food choices, and moving on to the next meal. Experiment to see what works for you. This isn't an easy process, however, it becomes less difficult over time.

"Don't cut out foods you know you'll binge on later. Include them in the meal plan."

Planning three meals a day begins with deciding *when* you're going to eat your meals. What are the best times to eat breakfast, lunch, and dinner? Try writing down meal times on your calendar or in your daily planner. You may have to accommodate work schedules or family members' plans, like taking kids to school or late-afternoon ball games. Make sure you have enough time for each meal and have easy access to foods, whether preparing the meal or eating out. Get in the habit of thinking about meal times and planning for them.

Choose foods you feel comfortable eating. Don't force yourself to eat something you're not ready to include in your meal plan, like foods that have felt threatening in the past. Also, don't cut out foods you know you'll binge on later. Include them in the meal plan.

Don't skip meals. If you do, get back on track by eating the very next meal. Eat whatever you want within those meal times and eat only what's on your plate. When you're finished, wait until the next meal to eat. If you get hungry in between, have a snack to tide you over.

The other approach to meal planning is to pick one meal and work on regulating it. For instance, if breakfast is your easiest meal, start there. Try to eat breakfast every day, initially choosing foods that you feel comfortable eating. Once eating breakfast becomes a habit, then add variety to the food choices. Choose foods you like to eat, but perhaps have limited in the past for fear you'd put on pounds. Breads, cereals, pancakes, waffles, French toast, egg dishes, fruits, and juices are all appropriate choices, as are sandwiches or leftover dinner items. It may take days, weeks, or months to become consistent with one meal. Once you master it, move on to the next meal, and then the third.

Avoid Deprivation

Allow yourself to eat whatever you want so that you don't feel deprived. This is one of the most common reasons for bingeing and eventual weight gain. If you currently eat or binge on desserts, sugar-sweetened foods, or salty snacks, and you want to continue eating them or feel you cannot give them up, include them in your meal plan. You may want to consider working on portion size right away if you feel distressed about eating large quantities of high-sugar, high-fat, or high-salt foods. Don't eliminate these foods from your life completely, however do begin to eat them in moderate amounts. Start to pare down the amount gradually so that it begins to approximate one serving size. If you eat more than what you would consider normal, that's okay. Begin over again at the next meal by eating a moderate amount.

At some point, you may want to consider abstaining from sugary or salty foods. Foods with sugar in them usually contain a high percentage of fat and are often used for bingeing. This is also true for high-salt/high-fat foods (e.g., potato chips and trail mix). Some people need to abstain from these kinds of foods completely, whereas others can eat them in moderation at meal time.

Another factor to consider is snacking between meals. Some people can handle a small snack, whereas others lose control when they start to snack, turning it into a binge, or grazing throughout the rest of the day. Decide for yourself whether you should only eat sweet and salty foods in moderation as part of a meal, or whether you can snack on them without overeating to allay your hunger until the next meal. Be honest with yourself about what works and what doesn't.

You may also be allergic or sensitive to some kinds of foods such as dairy products, nuts, certain fruits, vegetables, or grains. When you're in tune with your body, it will let you know what it likes, as well as what it may not be able to digest. For instance, if you're lactose intolerant and cannot handle dairy products, there are other sources of calcium ranging from dietary supplements to leafy green vegetables. You can get your protein from foods other than cheese, milk, or yogurt.

Moderation

The next step is to address moderation and the quality of the foods you eat. Use the palm of your hand as a gauge for portion size. When a food item looks like it's about the size of your palm, it's a moderate amount—about one serving. In terms of quality, make sure you select items from the five food groups (p. 62), to give yourself a variety of choices.

"If you eat what you want in moderation, incorporating healthy foods, you'll be eating a generally balanced diet."

The ratio of how much of each of these food groups to eat is important. Grains (bread, cereal, rice, and pasta) are the foods to eat the most of, then fruits and vegetables, then dairy and proteins (meat, poultry, fish, eggs, nuts, and beans—high in protein and carbohydrates), and finally a smaller amount of fat. Fats are necessary for building cell membranes, cushioning vital organs, providing insulation from cold weather, and maintaining menstruation and, thus, childbearing capabilities. The solution is finding a balance between the five food groups. However, don't stress out if you don't do it perfectly. If you eat what you want in moderation, incorporating healthy foods, you'll be eating a generally balanced diet.

As you begin feeding your body healthier kinds of foods, it will begin craving them. The healthiest foods are the least processed, meaning foods kept closest to their natural form. They're also naturally low in fat, sugar, and salt. The best foods are those prepared at home or in a restaurant using few additives and a small amount of fat in the cooking. Complex carbohydrates such as fruits, grains, vegetables, and beans can be as much as 65 percent of your daily intake. You can eat more complex carbohydrates during meals because they're low in fat. They become higher in fat when they're prepared with oils and butter. Dairy products and proteins are considered healthy when they have a low fat content. Carbohydrates and proteins contain four calories per gram, whereas fat has nine calories a gram, making it more than twice the caloric content of carbohydrates and proteins. When you eat fat, 98 percent of it goes directly into your fat cells and is stored there. Food doesn't lead to weight gain—fats, overeating, and a lack of moderate exercise do. People with no weight problems or food issues eat the same number of calories—and sometimes more calories—than overweight people. However, overweight people tend to get more calories from fat and fewer from complex carbohydrates.

Also, people who are dieting assume if they eat fat-free foods, they'll lose weight. Often, they don't consider the amount they eat, and actually overeat. You can gain weight when you eat fat-free cookies if you eat the whole box. That's because the total caloric content consumed in one sitting is extremely high. If you eat one or two servings of any food, you won't gain weight, and you don't have to stick to fat-free items. You can eat a variety of foods, as long as the portion size is moderate within mealtimes.

Remember, eating a variety of foods and making healthier choices are key components to maintaining a healthy weight. Try eating different kinds of foods during mealtimes. Experiment to see what works best for you.

Dehydration

Your body needs about six to eight glasses of water a day. It can easily become dehydrated, especially if you're purging, since both food and water are released through purging. If your body has been dehydrated for a period of time, and you then drink liquids, your hands and feet may swell. As your body does with food, it holds on to water to ensure it doesn't become dehydrated again. When you drink water consistently, your cells will discharge the excess liquid naturally, although it may take a few days or weeks for the body to release it.

Meal Preparation

Preparing regular meals can seem difficult in the beginning. If you feel overwhelmed by the very idea, do something else. There are many choices. You can buy frozen meals at the store, order restaurant takeout, or try some quick and easy home cooking. In the beginning, prepare or order only what you're going to eat. Making more food than you would eat in one sitting, with the intention of having leftovers, often leads to overeating. If you want a snack or dessert, buy only the amount you plan to eat, rather than keeping a stockpile in your cupboards. Do what is most comfortable and convenient for you. Don't push yourself to try things until you're ready. Over time, meal planning and preparation become easier, and you'll enjoy broadening your food choices.

Create an eating environment. Many people who struggle with food eat standing up, directly from the fridge, in front of the TV, or while driving. None of these styles allow you to gauge how much you're eating or feel as if you've had a satisfying meal. Eat only at the kitchen or dining room table. Set the table, sit down, eat slowly, chew each bite, taste the food, and don't read or watch TV while you eat.

Take time to notice the way you approach food. Pay attention to how the food tastes, how you experience it, how quickly you eat, how big each bite is, whether you put down utensils between bites, how long you take to finish the meal, and what you think about while you're eating. The slower you eat and the more you chew your food, the less you eat. You'll also enjoy the experience more. It takes about twenty minutes for your stomach to register fullness, so eating slowly allows your body to know when it's becoming full. In addition to paying attention to what and how you eat, this time can be used for sitting and thinking about personal things—career, relationships, goals, and dreams. Record in a journal any feelings that surface concerning food, eating, body image, or weight.

Notice how much time passes between your meals. Don't go more than four or five hours before eating again. When you eat a variety of foods regularly throughout the day, your body will become hungry every four or five hours. However, when you eat an all-carbohydrate meal, you may find yourself feeling hungry within two hours. That's why eating many kinds of food is recommended, including protein and some fats. Your body begs to be fed on a consistent basis. So, again, eat when you're hungry and stop when you're full.

"When you eat consistently, your metabolism has the opportunity to function at an optimum level and your fat cells shrink."

One huge benefit to eating every few hours is that your metabolism is less likely to slow down its burning of calories. When long stretches of time pass between meals, like eight or nine hours, your body assumes it's being starved. Your metabolic rate slows down to conserve energy and your fat cells prepare to store fat. When you eat consistently, your metabolism has the opportunity to function at an optimum level and your fat cells shrink. Be aware that your metabolism burns slower at night. Eat enough food for dinner without overeating so that you won't be snacking late into the evening.

If you find that you binge or begin grazing right after a meal, consciously put time between finishing the meal and eating again. This may mean just five minutes. Then stretch it to 10 minutes, 15 minutes, and so on. Eventually, you'll be able to prevent bingeing and grazing. This is discussed in more detail in "Frequency, Quantity, Quality: Preventing Unhealthy Eating Behaviors" (chapter 2–12).

Restaurant Eating

Eating in restaurants can be quite threatening, since many people think of restaurants as places to eat all the things they wouldn't normally eat. Simply remember, it's just like at home; you can eat anything you want when dining out, but keep the portions moderate. If you overeat, don't worry—it's only one meal. Get back on track the next meal.

Choose foods you like and choose variety. You can ask for salad dressings, mayonnaise, butter, or sour cream on the side of the dish rather than on top. This gives *you* control of what you eat, not the restaurant. If you really want to have something, have it. And remember, the least processed foods are the healthiest. Decide how much of an item you are going to eat and put the rest on another plate. Then eat only what's on your plate. When you're done with that, your meal is finished. This will ensure that you eat moderately, rather than letting the restaurant determine how much you'll eat.

Fast-food restaurants are often favorite stopping places for bingers and grazers. You can still eat at fast-food establishments, just approach dining in the same way as you do at other restaurants. Eat whatever you want, but in moderate amounts. You may, however, decide to make healthier food choices. Most fast-food restaurants offer lower-fat food items such as dishes made with skinless, grilled chicken. Or you might try modifying the existing menu by asking them to leave off the cheese, mayonnaise, or butter, and to add mustard, catsup, or hot sauce. You may never notice the difference. Also, order side salads—it's an easy way to get vegetables with your meals.

Elaine loved salsa and tortilla chips. Instead of eating dinner, she ate chips while watching TV, up until heading for bed. Although she usually ate a fairly balanced breakfast and lunch, she found herself grazing on chips just about every evening. The only time she ate a meal was when she went out with her boyfriend a couple of times a week. On the weekends, she sometimes had chips for lunch and dinner. Elaine's weight was also affected by how she ate. She wanted to lose the twenty pounds she gained since graduating from college, but hadn't been able to do so.

Eventually, she realized she was eating for emotional reasons as well as from habit. Eating kept her from thinking about her company's downsizing and how she felt stressed and anxious by her added responsibilities. The chips numbed and comforted her, yet changed nothing at work. She decided it was important to learn how to stop grazing and how to concentrate instead on dealing with her feelings.

When Elaine consulted me, her first question was, "Will I have to give up chips?" Once she learned she could have them, just not in the manner she was currently eating them, she thought what I proposed was doable. We worked on changing the way she approached the end of her day and evening. She ate a one-serving-size bag of chips for lunch along with a sandwich. Then, she ate the same size bag with dinner, but not as the main course. Eventually, she became more flexible about when she ate chips, and she didn't eat them at every meal.

She also needed something to help her de-stress once she got home. We designed an evening routine. Before preparing dinner, she would relax for twenty minutes, sometimes taking a bath while listening to her favorite tape. Other times, she would write in her journal about work experiences that were stressful. Then she prepared her meal and ate it. Once she was finished, she prevented herself from eating for the rest of the evening by spending time walking her dog, painting, reading, watching TV, or getting together with her boyfriend. Before she knew it, she went down a dress size, with less effort than dieting ever took.

Robin, unlike Elaine, ate only two small meals a day, fruit for breakfast and a store-bought low-fat frozen meal for dinner. The rest of the day she drank coffee to keep her awake and going. Sometimes when she was really hungry, she bought foods she normally wouldn't eat, chewed them up, and spit them out. She rationalized that at least she got to taste the forbidden foods without taking in any calories. Robin recognized this was a problem when she looked in her garbage can one day and saw a pile of sludge. She knew she needed to change what she was doing but was concerned about not feeling as powerful as she had when she withheld food.

Determined to change her habits, Robin contacted me for help. In our first meeting, her initial reaction was, "You mean I can eat anything I want and not get fat?" I told her that she could eat anything within moderation as long as she didn't overeat, ate only when hungry, and chose a variety of foods. I explained how restricting food negatively affected her metabolic function and fat storage. She was skeptical but open-minded.

With the aid of a registered dietitian, we designed meal plans and had her add foods to each meal. Robin started out by eating a small lunch. The first week she ate lunch two of the seven days. By the fourth week, she was eating soup and salad almost every day. Robin's biggest hurdle was adding variety. She knew the caloric content and fat grams of everything she ate. But other foods were unknowns. Over time, though, she added two pieces of toast with jam to breakfast and simple pasta or rice dishes to dinner. She has yet to eat vegetables, although she is eating some forbidden foods she had been spitting out. She has also cut back on the amount of coffee she drinks, from seven cups a day to three, and is drinking water and herbal teas.

Chewing and spitting out food was linked to feeling deprived of food, avoiding dealing with emotional upsets, and preventing weight gain. She also began exploring her feelings and learning better ways to handle them. As she has increased her ability to process feelings, she decreased her chewing-and-spitting behavior. Overall, Robin is feeling better, and she thinks it's great that she hasn't gained any weight.

Dealing With Emotions

When you begin to change your eating habits, a number of feelings can emerge. After all, food, or the lack of it, has been used to soothe and numb you for a very long time. It's normal for your feelings to come to the surface as you begin to heal. Use the "Face Your Feelings: Alternatives to Feed Your Emotions" (chapter 2-15) and "Part Three: Healing the Emotional Self and Mental Self" (chapters 3-1 to 3-10) to address any feelings that seem frightening or overwhelming.

Deal with food one day, or even one meal, at a time. Make it as easy and stress-free as possible when changing your behaviors. If you "blow it" at a meal, start over the very next meal. Don't wait until tomorrow or the following week to begin again. Each day builds on the previous one, and before you know it, you'll be more at ease with food and with meal planning.

Assignment: Explore what it means to begin planning your meals and eating three meals a day—which includes eating moderate amounts, making healthier food choices, avoiding deprivation by incorporating the foods you love, eating in restaurants or fast-food establishments, and facing your feelings. The following chapters will help you make the necessary changes in your eating and exercise habits.

2 - 4

Knock Down Barriers to Success: Overcome Obstacles That Prevent Change

On the road to changing your unhealthy eating habits, you're bound to face certain stumbling blocks...so be aware. One factor all harmful eating behaviors share is that

---

"Learning to reduce stress and handle tension more effectively will make it less likely that you'll turn to starving, bingeing, purging, or grazing to cope."

---

they're stress induced. These behaviors tend to reemerge or become more resistant to change during times of stress or tension. Learning to reduce stress and handle tension more effectively will make it less likely that you'll turn to starving, bingeing, grazing, or purging to cope. Following are some hurdles unique to each behavior that you might face when trying to make changes.

STARVING

The biggest struggle for people who starve is making sure they eat enough food throughout the day. Their problem is they don't eat enough food at mealtimes. When you starve yourself, you tend to deprive yourself of food by skipping meals, forcing yourself to eat extremely small portions of food, choosing only low-calorie foods such as vegetables, or eating foods with no fat. Start to change by eating three meals a day, even if it's only one food item at each meal. Then, slowly increase the amount and kinds of foods you eat. This means eating cereals, breads, pastas, rice, potatoes, beans, fruits, proteins, and dairy products. Your body needs a certain amount of fat. All bodies do. So, you need to avoid nonfat foods and start incorporating some fat into your meals. This means you can eat nuts, chips, and desserts as well (in moderation).

One of the biggest fears starvers have is overeating. But, you're less likely to overeat if you feed your body on a regular basis and give it enough food so that it does not feel hungry or deprived. Plan your meals, even if it's just a small amount of food at each meal. Ultimately, you may need to add snacks between meals to help you feed your body the amount of food it needs to function well.

"Don't try to change all your eating habits at once, that makes it too easy to revert back to starving."

If you're anorexic or need to gain weight, calculate how many calories a day you're eating. Remember, 1,200 is the minimum. Any amount below that doesn't allow your metabolism to function optimally and you begin to burn muscle. When your eating is regulated, you don't need to count calories; you can estimate how much you're eating by portion size. Eat regularly and moderately so that your body becomes accustomed to being fed. You will gain weight, however, it will increase gradually, level off, and stabilize at a healthy point.

Don't try to change all your eating habits at once, that makes it too easy to revert back to starving. Drink lots of liquids. Many people who starve themselves also limit how much they drink, believing that liquids make them heavier. They don't. You need liquids to prevent dehydration.

As you begin to refeed, you'll most likely notice many uncomfortable feelings arising. You'll need to find ways to deal with all the emotions that surface concerning food, eating, body image, and self-esteem (see "Face Your Feelings: Alternatives to Feed Your Emotions," chapter 2-15). As you begin to process your feelings, you'll notice they pass after a certain period of time. If you've lost a lot of weight and your behaviors are not changing with the help of this workbook, seek professional help.

Craig is a low-weight wrestler for his university. While on the high school wrestling team, he learned how to reduce his weight right before a match. He starved himself and drank few liquids to make sure he would be below his natural weight. After the competition, he found himself bingeing because he was so hungry. This led to temporary weight gain, which pushed him to fast for days before the next match. Once in a while, he used laxatives if he needed an extra boost. He also experienced emotional repercussions. He became moody and irritable when fasting and frustrated and depressed when bingeing. He was stuck in a cycle that was difficult to break.

He had been doing this on and off for four years, and felt he couldn't stop on his own. He contacted me for help. He knew he couldn't weigh his competing weight without taking extreme measures. We discussed his option of moving up one weight category to compete at that level. He was concerned that the coach would not allow that. However,

Craig convinced his coach that wrestling underweight was causing him great harm physically and emotionally. The coach agreed.

Craig then worked on changing his eating behaviors. To his surprise, he had become very accustomed to his diet/binge cycle. He thought he could give it up quite easily once he didn't have to lose weight for every competition. We focused on relearning how to eat three meals a day and how to make healthy food choices. He read books on how athletes eat to maintain energy and stamina, and he followed many of those guidelines. He also decided that he didn't want to give up eating donuts, so he ate them once or twice a week. Within six months, his weight stabilized at ten pounds higher than his starvation weight, and he was relatively binge free. Once in a while he slipped back into old patterns, but he always quickly got back on track. Best of all, he's a much better wrestler now that he has the strength to compete.

BINGEING AND PURGING

One of the hardest behaviors to give up is purging because those who purge strongly believe that it keeps off the weight. For your health's sake, you must stop the purging behavior. Not only is it dangerous, but it's not a method of weight control that you can use forever.

Cut down on your purging day by day. First, set a limit as to how many times a day you will engage in the behavior. If you purge four times a day, cut back to two times and stick with it. A few weeks later, cut down again. As you decrease the number of times you purge, you'll also need to address your bingeing. You purge because you've overeaten and fear you'll gain weight.

Work on planning meals and grouping foods into mealtimes. Eat three meals a day and snacks, if you need them, to prevent bingeing and purging. Mistakes and setbacks happen, so don't expect perfection. If you slip, get back on track the very next meal. As I mentioned in chapter 2–3, dehydration is a common side effect of purging. Drink liquids to hydrate your body again. Initially, your hands and feet may swell as your body eagerly holds on to all the liquids it receives. Over time, though, it will release excess liquids and the swelling will go down.

Various thoughts and feelings are bound to come up as you concentrate on changing your behavior. You'll need to address them so you don't return to either bingeing or purging to cope. If you're unable to stop the purging with the help of this workbook, seek professional help.

Amber and her friends loved to go on french fry runs. Every day after school they went to their favorite fast-food restaurant and ordered fries, hamburgers, and shakes. Since entering high school, Amber had learned all the tricks to keep off the weight she put on by bingeing—vomiting, laxatives, diuretics, and an occasional enema. So many of her friends had similar food problems and body image issues that Amber lost count. At first it was fun to go on these runs, but Amber got tired of feeling bad for days on end—eating lots of fatty foods and purging to prevent weight gain.

Amber decided to stop the bingeing and purging and told her mother about what she had been doing. When Amber and her mother met with me for the first time, Amber couldn't believe she would be able to eat hamburgers and fries and not get huge. The first step was to have her chart what she ate and when, noticing the times she felt the hungriest and which part of the month she craved certain kinds of foods. I helped her devise meal plans to follow. She picked foods she liked and included fries and hamburgers a couple of times a week.

Giving up purging was difficult in the beginning. Amber was sure she would gain weight. But as she gave up purging, she decreased her bingeing, substituted healthier foods, and started aerobic walking every other day. She also ate junk food whenever she really craved it. And she didn't gain weight. Amber has days when she slips back to the old behaviors, but they've become less often as time goes on.

Whenever Amber felt peer pressure to eat or look a certain way, she turned to the coping skills she learned in therapy. She talked more with her best friend and sometimes with her mother when she felt stressed out. She also started an ongoing journal of her experiences, thoughts, and feelings. These activities, along with exercise, were enough to help Amber deal with the strains of life in high school.

BINGEING AND GRAZING

The biggest hurdle for people who binge and graze is grouping foods into meals and eating only during mealtimes. Bingers tend to start eating whatever is around and don't stop until all the food is gone or the binge is interrupted. It's imperative that you plan your meals, curtail your eating when the food on the plate is gone, and wait for the next meal or snack to eat. First, work on consistently eating three meals a day. Second, address portion sizes and types of foods. This means eating moderate portions and choosing healthier kinds of food. Eating snacks and desserts can actually prevent bingeing and grazing. But be careful, they can also turn into overeating.

If you get hungry between meals and need to eat snacks, approach them as mini-meals. When the snack is gone, stop eating. Then wait until the next meal to eat again. You'll also need to explore the thoughts and feelings that arise during the periods between eating. This is initially difficult because you've been accustomed to using food to suppress unpleasant emotions. You'll need to learn how to experience your feelings without turning to food for comfort, consolation, or distraction. Use "Face Your Feelings: Alternatives to Feed Your Emotions" (chapter 2–15), to help with this process. Like the other unhealthy eating behaviors, if you are not able to stop the bingeing or grazing with this workbook, seek help.

Darlene ate a pound of chocolate every week. She swore up and down that she was addicted to chocolate and couldn't give it up. The more she ate, the more she craved. She ate it for every reason imaginable—when she was happy, upset, stressed, bored, or lonely. Not coincidentally, Darlene weighed 45 pounds more than she wanted to. She had tried all the latest magazine diets plus a number of weight-loss programs. For her last attempt at losing weight and curbing the chocolate obsession, she tried a store-bought vanilla-flavored liquid diet drink. This lasted a week. She always felt incredibly deprived and desperate for chocolate whenever dieting. She even dreamt about it.

Darlene consulted me as a last resort. Her husband had been urging her to seek help for a while, and when her last diet failed, she knew she couldn't stop what she was doing on her own. Once I explained why diets don't work, Darlene decided to give up dieting to see if the principles I proposed actually worked.

The first step was to help her set up daily meal plans that included many kinds of foods that are easily prepared. She read labels and kept fats and salts well below what she had in the past. She also ate chocolate, only less of it. Instead of buying a box of candy, she bought candy bars and ate them after lunch or dinner. Initially, she ate two or three in one sitting. Now she's eating one a day, and sometimes forgets to eat any at all.

She discovered that her body would tell her when she was hungry and when she was full and satisfied. She had been ignoring the messages for so long, that she didn't recognize what hunger and fullness felt like. Now she listens to her body and feeds it healthier foods. She started an exercise program three times a week—a step class at her local gym. With the combination of changing her eating habits and adding exercise, Darlene lost 35 pounds.

Darlene discovered that her husband Bill was having a difficult time with her changing. He was unconsciously sabotaging her new eating habits by bringing chocolate home. When she talked with him, he voiced discomfort with how assertive she had become in expressing her feelings, including how she felt about him and their relationship. They attended a few sessions with me, and we discussed better ways for them to communicate. Bill practiced being more expressive with his feelings and made a conscious effort to not bring chocolate into the house.

Assignment: Use the *Fears and Ambivalence* list to help you assess which factors stir up fear or ambivalence and stop you from changing unhealthy eating patterns.

FEARS AND AMBIVALENCE

Before taking steps to modify your eating behaviors, be aware of any fears and ambivalence that might get in the way of your making changes. You may fear you'll be unable to change, or you may be nervous about taking the necessary steps involved in

> *"Fears and feelings of ambivalence are a normal part of the healing process."*

learning new behaviors. Ambivalence means the inability to make a choice, or the simultaneous desire to do two opposite things. Maybe you really want to stop bingeing, but you also hate the thought of not eating whole cartons of butter pecan ice cream when you feel so inclined. These fears and feelings of ambivalence are a normal part of the healing process. You're asking yourself to alter behaviors that have helped you cope with a wide variety of emotions and stresses. However, the things you fear most almost never happen, and the feelings eventually pass. Once you recognize your fears and ambivalence and acknowledge them, you can deal with them. "Face Your Feelings: Alternatives to Feed Your Emotions" (chapter 2–15) and other applicable chapters in "Part Three: Healing the Emotional Self and Mental Self" (chapters 3-1 to 3-10) of this workbook will be helpful.

On the lines below, write down all your fears and feelings of ambivalence so that you know what you're facing.

1. _____

2. _____

3. _____

4. _____

5. _____

6. _____

7. _____

8. _____

9. _____

10. _____

11. _____

2 - 5

Reduce the Food Obsession: Twenty-Six Steps to Success

Below is a list of the different ways we've just discussed to make changes in how you approach mealtimes. The more you follow these suggestions on a regular basis, the less likely you'll struggle with food. The intent of these tips is to reduce your obsession with food. When you develop healthy habits, your behaviors become automatic and thoughts about food and eating actually decrease. Keep this list handy so you can refer to it often.

1. Eat three meals a day.

2. Don't skip meals.

3. Don't diet—find a way of eating you can commit to for the rest of your life without ever having to diet again.

4. Eat when hungry, stop when full.

5. Eat a minimum of 1,200 calories a day.

6. Don't count calories or calculate grams of fat, use portion size as a measure.

7. Plan meals either daily or weekly.

8. Select from the five food groups.

9. Eat moderate amounts of food (one to two servings) and make healthy food choices.

10. Don't deprive yourself of foods from your Bust "Bad" Foods Chart (p. 76). If you crave something, plan to eat it as part of a meal.

11. If you want to eat something sweet or salty, buy one serving size.

12. Snacking between meals is optional. If it turns into bingeing or grazing, snacks are not a good idea.

13. Once a meal is finished, wait until the next meal or snack to eat again.

14. When you get off track, eat normally at the next meal.

15. Take fifteen to twenty minutes to finish a meal; eat slowly and chew your food.

16. Eat at your kitchen or dining room table, not in front of the TV or refrigerator, or in your car.

17. Create a comfortable and pleasant eating environment.

18. When you go into a store with the intent to binge, give yourself the option of turning around and walking out empty-handed.

19. Drink six to eight glasses of water a day.

20. When you learn to eat normally, your body will stabilize at a weight that is healthy for you.

21. Weigh yourself once a week or less often until you can stop weighing yourself altogether.

22. To make permanent changes, alter one or two behaviors and stick with them until they become habits, then move on to the next behavior.

23. Make a daily commitment to work on eating behaviors.

24. Begin to deal with feelings that arise during the time between meals or before and after eating.

25. Do the best you can. There is no perfect eating.

26. Be patient.

Assignment: Circle the suggestions that you can use every day to help you alter your eating behaviors. Keep the list handy to remind yourself of the healthy habits you want to create.

2 - 6

Meals Made Easy:
Plan Ahead for Healthy Eating

Guidelines can be very helpful when making decisions about what to eat during mealtimes. A Food Guide Pyramid has been proposed by the United States Department of Agriculture (USDA) to help Americans eat healthily and moderately. Below is the diagram of that guide to help you understand how much to eat from each of the five food groups.

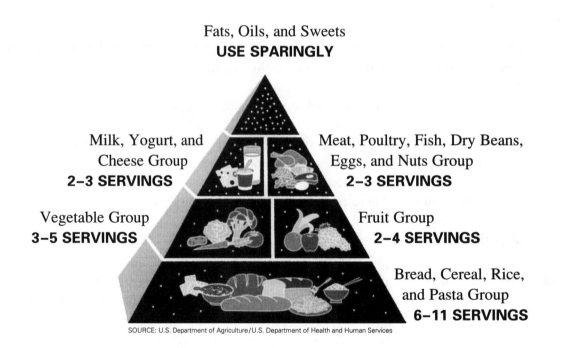

Fats, Oils, and Sweets
USE SPARINGLY

Milk, Yogurt, and
Cheese Group
2–3 SERVINGS

Meat, Poultry, Fish, Dry Beans,
Eggs, and Nuts Group
2–3 SERVINGS

Vegetable Group
3–5 SERVINGS

Fruit Group
2–4 SERVINGS

Bread, Cereal, Rice,
and Pasta Group
6–11 SERVINGS

SOURCE: U.S. Department of Agriculture/U.S. Department of Health and Human Services

The key to success in dealing with food and food issues is to figure out a way of eating that you can follow for the rest of your life without ever having to diet again. Consider the plan in this workbook to be a lifelong style of eating. The way you eat at this age is the way you can eat when you're 80 years old. Listed on the next page are the type and quantity of food choices the Food Guide Pyramid suggests.

MEAL PLAN

This is an ideal meal plan. Yours will be different, based on what you like to eat. Experiment to see what works best for you, and be sure to try various kinds of foods.

BREAKFAST	EXAMPLE
2 Breads/Cereal	2 Pieces of Toast with Honey
1–2 Fruits	1 Banana, 1 Cup of Juice
1 Protein (optional)	1 Egg
1 Dairy	1 Glass of Milk

SNACK	
1 Serving (Optional)	1 Pear, 1 Candy Bar, or 1 Bag of Chips

LUNCH	
2–3 Breads/Pasta/Rice	2 Breads for Sandwich
1–2 Fruits (Optional)	1 Apple
1–2 Vegetables	Lettuce & Tomato for Sandwich
1 Protein	2–3 oz. Tuna Fish
1 Dairy	1 Cup of Yogurt

SNACK	
1 Serving (Optional)	1 Cup of Raisins or 1 Cup of Trail Mix

DINNER	
2–3 Breads/Pasta/Rice	1 Cup Pasta
1–2 Fruits	1/4–1/2 Cantaloupe
1–2 Vegetables	1/2–1 Cup Tomato Pasta Sauce
1 Protein	2–3 oz. Beef for Pasta Sauce
1 Dairy (Optional)	1 Cup of Milk
1 Dessert (Optional)	1 Cup Rice Pudding

Some days you'll need a snack to tide you over until your next meal, other days you won't. There will also be days when you want a dessert after a meal, but not on other days. Remember to let your body be your guide as to what you hunger for, and choose moderate portions.

When planning meals, think about the variety of foods available to you. It's easy to limit your choices to "safe" or diet foods, meaning those that won't lead to weight gain. But try not to do that. You may tend to place other foods into one of two categories: binge foods or foods that taste awful. When certain foods don't taste good, it's often because you're unfamiliar with them or they aren't prepared in a tasty manner.

Many people think certain vegetables, fruits, beans, and whole-grain products have little or no taste—at least not when compared to the sugary, salty, or fatty foods so often chosen as binge foods. But, over time, your taste buds will become accustomed to the natural flavors in fruits, vegetables, grains, and beans. And the more you feed them to your body, the more you'll crave them.

Spend a little time learning how to prepare healthy foods. Bookstores devote numerous shelves to cookbooks filled with suggestions for simple ways to prepare foods in a healthful manner. Many restaurants also have healthy menu items.

To reduce your fat intake, you can buy special toppings to add to your healthy foods to improve the taste, such as lower-fat sour cream, cream cheese, and cheese; yogurt; butter sprinkles; and all-fruit jam. Plus, you can buy reduced-fat crackers, chips, cookies and desserts. However, you can gain weight if you binge on or consistently overeat any of these food items. Again, low- or nonfat items need to be part of an overall style of eating that includes a variety of foods, not just diet foods.

As I mentioned earlier, you can include foods that you previously binged on in your meals, just be sure to have them in one or two servings and with a meal. You may not want to eat them every day or all the time, but they can add variety to your meals, unless you find yourself bingeing on them again. Once these foods are no longer forbidden, you'll find it easier to eat them without overeating them.

The earlier menu example is what balanced meals look like. This is the ideal. No one eats this way all the time. You may be eating more at one meal than another or on one day than on others. And don't forget, eat when you're hungry and stop when you're full. You may also decide to have desserts with every meal to avoid bingeing. Everything is O.K.! You are on the path to discover how to eat meals again in a way that you can follow for the rest of your life.

Assignment: Here's where you learn how to plan your meals.

1. Use *Expanding Your Food Choices Chart* to list the foods you eat on a regular basis, the foods you don't eat, and forbidden foods. You'll want to increase the variety of foods you eat every day to prevent starving, bingeing, purging, or grazing.

2. Make daily or weekly meal plans using the *One-Week Menu Plan*. Remember, a balanced meal plan includes both nondiet foods as well as low- and nonfat items.

3. Take the meal plan with you when you shop for food.

4. On the days you eat out, stick to what you've decided to eat.

5. Incorporate into your meals a moderate amount (one or two servings) of the foods you know you'll binge or graze on. If you cannot eat certain foods because they're too threatening, give yourself permission to wait before adding them to your meal plan. Eat them when you're ready, not because you think you should.

6. Fill out the *Foods Eaten During Week* chart to see what you actually ate compared with what you had planned to eat. Notice where you're successful and the areas in which you struggle. Use this information to modify your approach, not beat yourself up. Make a daily or even moment-to-moment commitment to change your behaviors.

EXPANDING YOUR FOOD CHOICES CHART

List the kinds of foods you eat on a regular basis. Also, list the foods you don't eat, either because you don't like them or haven't tried them and think you wouldn't like them. Finally, list the foods you think are "bad," and therefore forbid yourself from eating.

Now, expand your choices. You will want to make your first list longer, and the other two shorter. For example, if you like sandwiches, think of all the kinds you can add to your "Foods You Eat" list. These can include: tuna, turkey, chicken, ham, cheese, roast beef, peanut butter and jelly, and burritos (chicken, beef, cheese, rice, or beans). If you're concerned about the amount of fat in sandwich fixings, choose reduced-fat meats, and low- or nonfat cheeses and mayonnaise. Add mustard, catsup, pickles, relish, lettuce, and tomatoes for flavor.

Try forbidden foods when you're ready to add them to your meal plan, and choose quantities that approximate one or two servings. Any more than that can lead to bingeing or grazing, which will land the food right back on the "bad" list again.

FOODS YOU EAT	FOODS YOU DON'T EAT	FORBIDDEN FOODS
1.		
2.		
3.		
4.		
5.		
6.		
7.		
8.		
9.		
10.		
11.		
12.		
13.		
14.		
15.		
16.		

ONE-WEEK MENU PLAN

To plan meals, either daily or weekly, make a list of foods you can buy and prepare or purchase as takeout.

	BREAKFAST	LUNCH	DINNER	SNACKS
Day 1				
Day 2				
Day 3				
Day 4				
Day 5				
Day 6				
Day 7				

FOODS EATEN DURING WEEK

List the foods you actually ate during the week. This will give you an idea where you're successful and where to fine-tune meal plans.

	BREAKFAST	LUNCH	DINNER	SNACKS
Day 1				
Day 2				
Day 3				
Day 4				
Day 5				
Day 6				
Day 7				

2 - 7

Chart Your Way to Change: Understanding Your Eating Behaviors

Until you understand your eating behaviors, you won't be able to change them. Become consciously aware of what you're doing with food by listing what foods you eat, when you eat them, and what feelings, if any, are leading you to eat. This will help you discover specific patterns and habits, and you'll be surprised to learn at what times you eat the most food, when you eat the least, which meals are hardest to plan, what kinds of foods you select most often, which foods you avoid, how much food you consume throughout the day, and why you ate—whether you were physically hungry or used food to cope with your emotions.

Dan's biggest hurdle was walking past the candy machine at work and not buying anything. As he arrived every morning, he would buy three or four candy bars. A slow weight gain had led him to feel guilty when he ate candy. He felt frustrated at not being able to stop what he was doing, even though he could see the problem so clearly. It was as if another part of him took over and walked him to the machine and bought the candy without his consent.

After months of trying to stop on his own, Dan contacted me. We explored what was compelling him to eat so much candy: part was habit, part was that he liked the taste of nuts and caramel, and part was to calm himself in the middle of a hectic day. After Dan charted his current eating behaviors, it was apparent that he snacked on candy bars between two and four in the afternoon. Meals weren't the problem; he ate three fairly balanced meals. It was the snacking on candy that was causing the weight gain.

We devised a simple yet effective plan to deal with his dilemma, arriving at three solutions. The first was to walk a different route through the building. The second was to buy only one candy bar and either eat it with lunch or as a mid-afternoon snack. And the third was to use his afternoon break for relaxation and meditation, which he learned in his yoga class. Dan found that he could live with all three options. Plus, he gradually became less tense in general and felt his quality of work life improve. He didn't feel deprived and lost weight without dieting.

Assignment: Keep track of your eating behaviors for a minimum of a week.

1. Use the *Current Eating Behaviors Chart* to help you identify which areas will be easiest for you to tackle and which will be the hardest. Address the easiest ones first; you're more likely to succeed that way. When you feel confident with your initial changes, move on to the harder ones. If you wish to see the changes in your behaviors over time, do your charting for longer periods. Simply paying attention to the amount of food you've consumed helps you to decrease the amount you eat.

2. See if you can make the connection between starving, bingeing, purging, or grazing and your emotions. Once you discover the emotions over which you eat or deny yourself food, you can address your emotions in a healthier way.

CURRENT EATING BEHAVIORS CHART

List the time of day you ate, what you ate and drank, the amount consumed, and why you ate—be it for physical hunger or emotional reasons.

TIME OF DAY	FOODS AND LIQUIDS CONSUMED	AMOUNT CONSUMED	WHY YOU ATE

2 - 8

Physical Hunger vs. Emotional Hunger: How to Recognize the Difference

It's often difficult to differentiate between physical and emotional hunger when your eating is inconsistent. Once you begin to eat regularly throughout the day, your body starts to give you clues to its degree of physical hunger. The rest of the sensations you interpret as hunger pangs are emotional.

Physical Hunger: Signs of physical hunger are distinct from those caused by emotional hunger. The most frequent signs of physical hunger include:

- Growling stomach
- Empty stomach
- Headache
- Dizziness
- Fatigue
- Irritability
- Moodiness

Emotional Hunger: This feels different than physical hunger, since it's emotionally based. Some of the kinds of emotional experiences and thought processes that lead to eating include:

- Depression
- Anxiety
- Boredom
- Loneliness
- Sadness
- Anger

- Frustration

- Internal emptiness

- Food as a reward for a successful experience

- Food as a punishment for being bad

Have you ever been aware of uncomfortable feelings and found yourself reaching for food as a way of dealing with them? That's one of the biggest indicators of emotional hunger. A second indicator is wanting to eat again within two hours of consuming a filling, balanced meal.

When you eat on a regular basis throughout the day, your body is able to send you messages about hunger and fullness. You'll feel physically hungry prior to you next scheduled meal. The rest of the feelings you experience are emotional hunger. Once your eating becomes consistent, food will no longer mask your emotions. You will be more aware of your feelings and you will have the opportunity to process them.

Eric ate one meal a day—a huge dinner. He claimed it was the only way he could weigh close to what he wanted to weigh. He let himself get so wrapped up in his work that he would forget to eat. If he became light-headed or drowsy, he'd drink a Coke or two, which gave him an energy boost until the end of the day. By three in the afternoon, Eric felt irritable and short-tempered, but he pushed through until five, when he left work. Then he went to the gym to play racquetball for an hour before heading home to help his wife prepare dinner for the family. He always had two servings of everything, and then felt utterly satisfied.

He couldn't manage to lose the 15 pounds he'd been wanting to shed for years. His wife urged him to eat more during the day and less at night. He was sure he would weigh even more if he did that. Because Eric ate only once every 24 hours, his body alternated between feeling full and famished. His body was retaining the 15 pounds as a cushion in case a real famine came along.

Eric found his way to my office when he heard about my diet-free solution to weight management. He really wanted to lose those 15 pounds, but had a difficult time believing that spreading out his daily intake into three meals would lead to weight loss, until he put the plan into action. His wife helped him; they fixed breakfast together and he took lunch to work. Sure enough, within six months the weight came off. And his hunger-induced mood swings all but disappeared.

Assignment: Use the *Physical and Emotional Hunger Chart* to list your hunger signals. By distinguishing between the two, you can respond by either feeding your body when physically hungry or attending to your feelings when emotionally hungry.

PHYSICAL AND EMOTIONAL HUNGER CHART

Make separate lists of your physical and emotional hunger signals. Once you recognize the difference, you'll be able to respond by either feeding your body or attending to your emotions.

PHYSICAL HUNGER	EMOTIONAL HUNGER
1. _____	1. _____
2. _____	2. _____
3. _____	3. _____
4. _____	4. _____
5. _____	5. _____
6. _____	6. _____
7. _____	7. _____
8. _____	8. _____
9. _____	9. _____
10. _____	10. _____
11. _____	11. _____
12. _____	12. _____
13. _____	13. _____
14. _____	14. _____
15. _____	15. _____
16. _____	16. _____
17. _____	17. _____
18. _____	18. _____

2 - 9

Bust the "Bad" Foods Myth: Eat Anything You Want, Within Reason

It's true. There are no "bad" foods. You can eat anything you want. However, eating anything and everything all the time will lead to weight gain, which is why a "bad" foods list was created in the first place. Diet plans and programs rely on the concept of

---

"If you include 'bad' foods in your way of eating, you'll be less likely to feel deprived and, likewise, less likely to use them for bingeing."

"good" and "bad" foods. Diets promote eating restrictively to create weight loss without addressing how to eat foods that traditionally have been considered binge foods. If you include these items in your way of eating, you'll be less likely to feel deprived and, likewise, less likely to use them for bingeing. People who don't have issues with food or weight eat whatever they want in moderation. They may eat more than they desire at times, but it doesn't turn into a bingeing/purging, bingeing/starving, grazing, or starving cycle.

You'll want to learn how to eat all kinds of foods without feeling threatened by them. "Bad" foods only have control over you if you give them that power. You're the one choosing what you'll eat—the food doesn't decide for you. Take some chances with eating forbidden foods in moderate amounts, and see the fear melt away.

Gretchen thought she could never eat pizza because of all the cheese. She was overly concerned about the fat content in foods and fastidiously calculated fat grams. She feared she'd gain weight, even though her weight was considered normal. So, in spite of her love of pizza, she avoided it.

Yet pizza was one of the foods Gretchen really wanted to eat again, so we discussed ways she could do that. She began by ordering vegetarian pizza with light cheese. She was worried her kids wouldn't eat a pizza that didn't have gobs of cheese, but they loved it, and so did she. She allowed herself to eat two pieces, then her family ate the rest. Gretchen realized that two slices, along with a salad, made a decent meal. She's still concerned about fat grams, but is consciously stopping herself from calculating the fat in everything she eats.

Assignment: Discover that there truly are no "bad" foods. Use the *Busting "Bad" Foods Chart* to list forbidden foods and how you can work them into your meal plan. Here's where you'll learn how to include foods you've been avoiding because you fear bingeing on them or gaining weight. You don't have to do it all at once. In fact, it's easier to start with the least threatening foods and then move on to the more threatening ones. There may be some foods that are just too scary to include, and it may take a while before you can eat them comfortably. That's fine. Go as slowly or as quickly as you need to.

BUSTING "BAD" FOODS CHART

List your "bad" foods in order of least threatening to most threatening and note how you will work them into your meal plan.

"BAD" FOODS	MEAL PLAN
1.	
2.	
3.	
4.	
5.	
6.	
7.	
8.	
9.	
10.	
11.	
12.	
13.	
14.	
15.	
16.	
17.	
18.	

2 - 10

Reverse Eating Rituals:
Face Food in New Ways

Eating rituals are behaviors you repeat (over and over again) in the same set manner to prevent weight gain. They become compulsive and automatic, as if they contain some

---

"Eating rituals keep you obsessed with food.
They signify being stuck in repetitive and
sometimes destructive eating habits."

---

magical quality that will help you with weight management. In reality, however, eating rituals keep you obsessed with food. They signify being stuck in repetitive and sometimes destructive eating habits. You must address these rituals by working toward flexible and healthy eating behaviors. When you let go of them, you'll be less focused on what you eat and how much you weigh. Again, this takes time and commitment. The first step is giving yourself permission to try new ways of approaching food.

Eating rituals might include:

- Counting bites

- Counting the number of times each bite is chewed

- Separating foods on the plate into distinct piles

- Eating only one kind of food at a time

- Making food last as long as possible

- Eating so quickly that you don't taste the food

- Chewing food and spitting it out instead of swallowing it

- Bingeing on "junk food" and dieting on "healthy food"

- Waiting until evening to eat your first meal

- Eating "forbidden" foods in secret

Paula considered herself a picky eater. She told her friends she could eat only certain things because she was "allergic" to many foods. Secretly, though, she ate those foods when no one was around. When Paula went out to restaurants with her friends, they were forced to choose places where she could find something to eat. When she ate at home with her parents, she prepared her own nonfat foods, refusing to eat what they did. She separated the foods on her plate so they didn't touch, finishing one pile before going on to the next.

Paula's friends and family stopped commenting on her eating habits because it caused conflict. She knew her style of eating was becoming more odd as time went on, and she felt depressed more often than not. Finally, she developed the ritual of sucking on food to make it last as long as possible. She reasoned that by doing this she would eat less, not gain weight, and not feel hungry after a meal that didn't satisfy her. Paula felt more obsessed with food than ever before and was frustrated at how much time she spent planning what she would eat.

When Paula consulted me for help, she was surprised to hear that the way she was eating was working against her, making her more obsessed with food, and that it would get worse if she continued to eat that way. We devised a game plan she could live with. First, she had to stop eating foods in secret and instead incorporate them into her meals every day. This added more of a variety—nonfat foods and regular items. She also tried to eat some of the things her family prepared. Instead of eating one food at a time from her plate, she built a mountain on her spoon, a layering of each food. And she made an effort to swallow the food instead of sucking on it.

Paula also cut down on the number of times per week she weighed herself, eventually weighing in once a month. This reduced her drive to weigh a certain weight. She became less focused on her body and found that her depression lifted. When she had a difficult day, she'd go back to the original plan and follow it. As time passed, Paula realized how much freer she felt and experienced a greater sense of control over her life.

Assignment: Use the *Eating Rituals Chart* to list your ritualistic behaviors, why you do them, and the healthy habits with which you envision replacing your rituals. Start with one ritual at a time, exchanging it with a more moderate, balanced behavior. Because ritualized habits are linked, when you begin to change one, the others are more easily altered.

EATING RITUALS CHART

List your current eating rituals, why you do them, and the healthy habits you envision yourself replacing them with.

RITUALS	WHY YOU DO THEM	HEALTHY EATING HABITS
1. _____		_____
2. _____		_____
3. _____		_____
4. _____		_____
5. _____		_____
6. _____		_____
7. _____		_____
8. _____		_____
9. _____		_____
10. _____		_____
11. _____		_____
12. _____		_____
13. _____		_____
14. _____		_____
15. _____		_____
16. _____		_____
17. _____		_____
18. _____		_____

2 - 11

Recognize Your Danger Zones:
Options to Food Abuse

Eating behaviors often feel like they come out of nowhere. Once the thought of food enters your mind, the desire to eat increases, making it seem impossible for you not to act on the impulse. You immediately develop severe tunnel vision, and you can't think of doing anything other than eating. It starts to feel like a losing battle.

"Once you've identified your danger zones, the situations that create the behaviors become much less threatening."

By keeping track of your behaviors, you can develop an awareness of when, where, and why you do what you do. Once you've identified your danger zones, the situations that create the behaviors become much less threatening. Then, you can learn to alter these circumstances or avoid them completely by making conscious choices to do something other than eat.

The key is to make different decisions. Even when you feel compelled to engage in unhealthy eating behaviors, you always have the choice to do something else. You do this by creating a list of things to do instead of bingeing, purging, grazing, or starving. The list can include behaviors like walking out of the store before you purchase something, buying one serving size instead of a whole box or bag of food, throwing the remainder of your meal away once you've finished, taking a walk or calling someone instead of purging, or eating everything you placed on your plate so you don't starve yourself. You keep the list in a place where you can easily read it. This can mean posting it on your refrigerator, placing it in your wallet, taping it to your TV set, or keeping it in your schedule book. You make a daily commitment to yourself that you will be consciously aware of your behaviors and will pull the list out when you need it. In the beginning, you won't necessarily choose from your list all the time, however, as you give yourself the opportunity for change and take the chance, it will become easier and more automatic.

Below are examples of the most common danger zones for the majority of people. See which ones apply to you.

1. Bingeing after work or school

2. Eating in the car

3. Stashing food in drawers and sneak-eating when no one is looking

4. Looking for fast food restaurants or convenience stores while driving

5. Shopping when hungry

6. Shopping without a grocery list

7. Buying too much food to eat in one sitting

8. Buying ice cream or liquids with the intent to purge

9. Eating less than 1,200 calories a day

10. Counting calories and/or calculating grams of fat in foods

11. Limiting food choices

12. Skipping meals to lose weight

13. Eating only vegetables or salads for a meal

14. Eating only desserts for a meal

15. Giving yourself permission for one last binge, then swearing you'll never do it again

16. Bingeing today because you're starting a new diet tomorrow

17. Spending hours planning a binge and/or purge

18. Weighing yourself every day or many times a day

19. Trying the latest fad diet with the intent to lose weight quickly

20. Exercising excessively

21. Ignoring your feelings

22. Isolating yourself from others

Wendy had her routine down. When her roommates left for class in the morning, she stayed at home to study and snuck out the stash of cookies that she kept hidden under her bed. Wendy deliberately chose late morning and early afternoon classes so she'd have time at home alone to eat. She didn't keep sweets in the kitchen because she didn't want her roommates to know that she ate a bag of cookies every day or so. She almost got caught a while ago when one of her roommates came home early, but she quickly threw the food into her sweater drawer before anyone saw her. Wendy completely forgot about the half-eaten cookies until she pulled her sweater out a few months later and it was dusted with cookie crumbs.

Wendy came to see me to understand why she binged and how to stop it. I pointed out that there was a strong link between how she felt and what she ate. For example, when she missed her boyfriend who was in school 200 miles away, she reached for cookies to help ease the ache. She was surprised to discover this connection between feelings and food. Once she developed ways to handle her emotions by choosing other behaviors aside from eating, she rarely binged. She created a list of options and carried it in her notebook. The list included not storing cookies in her bedroom, buying one serving of cookies if she wanted to have them, eating them in the open, talking about her feelings to others instead of reaching for food, walking in the mountains, and writing in her journal about daily events. Eating cookies became very satisfying once she removed the emotional reasons for wanting them.

Assignment: Examine what situations make you more vulnerable to starving, bingeing, purging, or grazing. Use the *Danger Zones Chart* to identify these situations and the different options you might try instead of giving in to your old, familiar eating habits.

DANGER ZONES CHART

List your danger zones and write down some options you might try instead of engaging in these behaviors.

DANGER ZONES	OPTIONS
1.	
2.	
3.	
4.	
5.	
6.	
7.	
8.	
9.	
10.	
11.	
12.	
13.	
14.	
15.	
16.	
17.	
18.	

2 - 12

Frequency, Quantity, Quality:
Preventing Unhealthy Eating Behaviors

In order to heal, you must first learn to delay, and eventually prevent, destructive and unhealthy eating behaviors. To do so, consider these three important factors:

1. How much time is there between your meals or eating episodes?

2. How much food do you eat?

3. What kinds of food do you eat?

Each of the behaviors I discuss in this workbook has its own unique trouble spots that need to be addressed in specific ways.

STARVING

When you starve yourself, you let too much time elapse between meals and you don't eat enough at one sitting. The first step toward changing this is to pay attention to how often you eat. If you eat two meals or less during the day, increase them to three. The best way

> *"Your goal needs to be to eat no fewer than 1,200 calories a day. Anything under that and the body believes it's in a starvation state and functions in a crisis mode."*

to set this pattern is to eat every four or five hours. This will ensure that you're actually getting three meals a day. Initially, you may need to set a timer to beep every four hours, or place markers in your schedule book at four-hour intervals until the new meal schedule becomes a habit.

The next step is to address the quantity of food you eat during each meal. You will need to eat enough to help maintain your weight (if you are not underweight) or gain weight (if you are underweight). Your goal needs to be to eat no fewer than 1,200 calories a day. Anything under that and the body believes it's in a starvation state and functions in a crisis mode. Work up to eating more calories by slowly adding one food item at a time to each meal.

Last, look at the quality of food you eat. Pick a variety of foods from all the food groups. And don't limit yourself to low-calorie food items like vegetables or store-bought diet foods. Start adding foods that you have enjoyed in the past. Each time you add a new item, you are moving toward eating balanced meals. As I mentioned previously, a number of feelings may arise when you regulate your eating. Use "Face Your Feelings: Alternatives to Feed Your Emotions" (chapter 2-15) to help you deal with any issues that make you uncomfortable.

Ellie starved herself. One year ago, she began dieting and eventually reached a point where she was eating very little food. No breakfast, an apple and five nonfat crackers for lunch, and four rice cakes with a large vegetable salad drowned in nonfat Italian dressing for dinner were all she would allow herself. Not surprisingly, she lost weight. She felt hungry all the time and realized she was creating serious problems by eating so little. She decided, with my help and that of a registered dietitian, to make changes in what she ate. Her initial goal was to add one food item to each meal: a piece of toast for breakfast, a cup of chicken or vegetable/beef soup for lunch, and a baked potato for dinner.

Due to her severely restrictive dieting, Ellie's metabolism had slowed down. As she ate more food, her metabolism began to burn at a higher rate. Each week, Ellie added food to her meal plans until she was eating 1,400 calories a day. She also stopped counting calories and paid more attention to planning her meals so that she'd eat enough food at each meal.

In the beginning, Ellie feared she would gain weight or eat uncontrollably and, therefore, was afraid of food in general. In spite of this, at every meal she faced her fear and encouraged herself to eat what she had planned. Within a few months, she was less afraid because her weight gain was slow and she didn't binge. She needed to gain 18 pounds, which took her six months. She learned to accept the fact that she couldn't weigh what she had weighed while starving herself because the weight and starving behaviors weren't healthy.

Today, Ellie is working on accepting her body at its new weight. To help achieve this, she avoids weighing herself and trusts that by eating regularly and moderately, her weight will not increase above her goal, and it hasn't.

BINGEING AND GRAZING

People who binge and graze are the opposite of those who starve. They make unhealthy food choices, eat too much food at one sitting, and don't wait long enough between eating episodes. If you fall into this category, the first step toward changing is to group foods into separate meals with at least four hours in between them. This sets up the habit of

---

"If you really want to binge on some food item, save it for your next meal."

---

eating three meals a day. When you feel the urge to binge or graze between meals, delay the behavior. Even five minutes of delaying a binge after thinking about it can be monumental. Your goal is to increase the time between the thought of a binge and actually going through with it. Eventually, you'll learn to delay long enough that you'll actually avoid bingeing or grazing. If you really want to binge on some food item, save it for your next meal. This way you're not depriving yourself of the food, just structuring it into your mealtime.

As you work at changing your behavior, also consider how much food you're eating at a meal and the kinds of foods you choose. Remember to use the palm of your hand as a guide for portion size and to include a variety of foods at each meal. This will help you to eat more healthily and more moderately. As with any change in behavior, certain feelings may emerge between mealtimes. Use the "Face Your Feelings: Alternatives to Feed Your Emotions" (chapter 2-15) to help you deal with any uncomfortable emotions that arise.

Caroline was a compulsive overeater, regularly choosing high-fat, high-salt, and high-sugar foods for her meals and binges. She kept those foods around the house "for her kids and husband," yet she ate almost all of them. They complained that there was never anything left over for them. She was clear that she had a problem—a slow weight gain since her last child was born three years ago was concrete evidence. She also noticed feeling more "blue." Her husband even commented on how her moods had changed since she gained weight.

By the time Caroline came to see me, she was feeling out of control with her eating and distressed about her weight. She didn't know how she could keep sweets and chips in the house for her family without eating them herself. She made a list of foods she could have in the house while learning to eat more healthily, including snack foods for herself and her family. I told her she could eat those items, in one-serving-size portions and as part of her meal, along with other foods that are naturally low in fat, salt, and sugar such as fruits, vegetables, grains, and beans. She found simple recipes that used a variety of foods she and her family liked. If she wanted to binge but wasn't hungry, she looked at what was making her turn to food. She eventually got pretty good at not reaching for Fritos and, instead, dealing with her emotions. Caroline was thrilled when the weight slowly came off, and her "blue" moods began to lift.

PURGING

Most purging is induced right after bingeing. To heal, you must reduce and eventually eliminate the number of times you purge. You can do this by placing time between the binge and the purge. First, be aware of when and why you purge. The urge to purge will pass if you give it enough time. So, create space between the thought of purging and actually doing it. Start by delaying for just five minutes. Then, each time you binge, put more time between the bingeing and the purging. Eventually, you'll put enough time between them that the intense desire will pass and you will have prevented a purge.

You also need to address bingeing. Read the earlier section on bingeing for help. You will learn that you must deal with feelings that you've been avoiding through bingeing and purging. If you don't deal with them, you may return to the old familiar behaviors. These feelings will pass if you give them the chance.

"You'll find that if you refrain from bingeing and purging, your weight is likely to stay the same or even decrease."

Try making a list of three things to do before opting to purge. For example, you could take a walk, then take a shower, then brush your teeth. You'll notice that the desire to purge will decrease as you pursue these other activities. Again, use "Face Your Feelings: Alternatives to Feed Your Emotions" (chapter 2-15) to help you make choices other than purging.

For purgers, as for others fighting the food issues battle, the biggest fear is weight gain. That's why purging is used as a method of weight control. But you'll find that if you refrain from bingeing or purging, your weight is likely to stay the same or even decrease.

Lila vomited after overeating almost every day for over a year. She first figured out how to purge after eating too much at Thanksgiving dinner. Purging seemed like the ultimate solution to any weight gain she might have from overeating. But she soon recognized that purging was making things worse. She became more obsessed with food and her weight was higher than ever before. An annual physical examination prompted her to address her behavior; she was afraid she was doing irreparable damage to her body.

Lila's physician referred her to my office. Lila was concerned about not being able to stop what she was doing. I suggested she start by putting time between her bingeing and purging, the thought of bingeing and the behavior, and the thought of purging and the behavior. The goal was to delay a binge or a purge and eventually prevent it. If she reduced her bingeing, she would reduce the desire to purge. She began delaying a few minutes, moving up to ten, then fifteen, then thirty minutes. She created a list of activities she could do instead of bingeing and/or purging, depending on where she was able to stop the cycle. Her list included walking her dog, calling at least two people from her support group, and writing in her journal. Some days were harder than others, but over time, she was able to reduce her purging to once a week. She's continuing with her plan to reduce the purging completely.

Also, Lila examined what she ate and why. We devised ways for her to plan meals and pick foods that didn't leave her feeling deprived, but also didn't create weight gain. Another thing Lila had to learn was how to deal with stresses and uncomfortable feelings without turning to food. With the help of therapy and a support group, she discovered she could sit through her feelings and she wouldn't die. Her friends were very supportive when she needed to call and talk about what she was experiencing. Writing in her journal also helped. Most of the time Lila is now able to tolerate her feelings and not turn to food.

Assignment: Use the *Delaying and Preventing Behaviors Chart* to help you delay or prevent unhealthy eating behaviors on a daily basis. The chart provides a place to list the kinds of food you eat, the time between each episode of eating, and your thoughts and feelings at the time. The goal is to increase the time between the moment you think about bingeing, purging, or grazing and when you actually do it. Eventually, you'll stop yourself. For starvers, the goal is to reduce the time between eating episodes. You'll also want to eat appropriate amounts of food and make healthier food choices. If you revert to old behaviors, get back on track the very next meal. Don't wait until tomorrow or Monday to start. Give yourself weeks or even months to work on changing your behaviors. Though the changes are often small, they build on each other so that eventually you will get to where you want to be.

DELAYING AND PREVENTING BEHAVIORS CHART

Make a list of what you ate at each meal; how long you delayed bingeing, purging, starving, or grazing; whether you prevented the behavior altogether; and your thoughts and feelings.

Meal	15 min.	30 min.	1 hr.	1.5 hrs.	2 hrs.	2.5 hrs.	3 hrs.	3.5 hrs.	4 hrs.	4+ hrs.	Thoughts and Feelings
Breakfast											
Snack											
Lunch											
Snack											
Dinner											

2 - 13

Get Moving!:
Exercise Will Change Your Weight the Easy Way

One of the most important components of the healing process is exercise. Just as you might first find it difficult to eat moderately and regularly, you might also find it hard to exercise. Most likely, you're now exercising to some degree—it may be too much or it may be too little. Most people don't exercise enough. Only 20 percent of Americans exercise three times a week for twenty minutes. Eighty percent exercise less than that. Neither over- nor underexercising will provide you the extraordinary benefits that come with exercising appropriately.

"Exercise readjusts the setpoint of the weight-regulating mechanism to lower the body's weight naturally."

Endorphins: One of the best by-products of exercise are endorphins, chemicals that are released from the brain as a result of sustained physical activity. They are released into the body within five to ten minutes of beginning to exercise, and they act like natural opiates, creating a sense of well-being and calmness, and alleviating depression.

Insulin: Insulin is also affected by exercise. An essential hormone, insulin allows cells in the body to absorb and burn sugar. When your system has excess insulin, the body converts sugar in the bloodstream to fat and then stores it. Exercise increases the cells' ability to use sugar, which keeps it from turning into fat.

Metabolic Rate: Physical activity also increases the body's metabolic rate, which means you will burn more calories throughout the day. Exercise readjusts the setpoint of the weight-regulating mechanism to lower the body's weight naturally. It's almost like telling your fat cells to get smaller because the body no longer needs that amount of fat. The body likes being mobile. So, in general, people who are sedentary weigh more than people who are active.

Fat-Burning Enzymes: Another benefit exercise offers is that when the body builds muscle through physical activity, it in turn utilizes certain enzymes to burn fat. So the more muscle the body has, the more fat it will burn on an ongoing basis.

Muscle Mass: To burn fat, the body needs muscle. Fat is removed from fat cells to be burned in the muscles and used for energy. When a diet is too restrictive, lean muscle is lost as well as fat. Then, when muscle mass decreases, the body's ability to burn fat lessens. Therefore, exercise and healthy eating combined allow the body to build muscle mass, which in turn, burns fat.

Cardiovascular: Aerobic exercise reduces major risk factors associated with heart disease, diabetes, and even some kinds of cancers. Exercise does this by thickening the heart muscle and pumping more oxygenated blood, keeping blood vessels clear of plaque, lessening the risk of dangerous blood clots, lowering blood pressure, raising healthy HDL cholesterol levels, and speeding up the transport of waste in the intestinal tract so the colon isn't irritated.[1]

Hormones: For women, exercise limits the amount of estrogen produced, which means that exercise may protect against estrogen-sensitive cancers including breast, endometrial, and ovarian.

When you create your exercise program, you should consider three very important components. The first is intensity. Low-intensity exercise won't affect fat storage. Muscle toning exercises, for example, do just what their name implies. However, they don't affect fat storage. High-intensity exercise doesn't burn fat either. What it does is use up sugar in the system. So, if your breathing is too hard and labored when you exercise, you're probably burning sugars rather than fats. Moderate intensity at a consistent pace is best because it burns fat and builds muscles at the same time.

When assessing the degree of intensity of your exercise program, pay attention to your pulse rate. Remember, if you exercise either too hard or not hard enough, your body doesn't receive the maximum benefits from the activity. When you exercise, your pulse rate should increase quickly and then level off. For beginners, the exercise pulse rate should be 70 percent of their maximum; for people who have been exercising a while, the pulse rate should be 80 percent of maximum.

How do I measure this, you might ask? First, learn what your resting pulse rate is by holding your wrist and counting the pulse for ten seconds. Multiply this number by six to get your pulse rate for one minute. Then double that number and you'll have your maximum pulse rate (100 percent). For example, if your resting pulse rate is 60, your 100 percent maximum pulse rate is 120. Seventy percent of 120 is 84, and 80 percent is 98.

[1] Simon, H. *Conquering Heart Disease.* New York: Little, Brown, 1994.

Measure your pulse three to four minutes into the exercise routine. After you calculate your pulse rate, continue to exercise. Adjust the level of activity to either increase or decrease your pulse rate. You only need to measure your exercise pulse rate a few times to know what your body feels like when it's exercising at an optimum level.

> *"Pick an activity you enjoy, since people rarely stick to exercise regimens that are too complicated, difficult, or boring."*

The second component is quantity—the amount of time per workout. The average workout needs to be 20 to 60 minutes long. Anything less and you're not allowing your body to get the full benefits of increasing your metabolic rate, building muscle, and releasing endorphins. Anything more than 60 minutes and you're setting yourself up for potential injury, strains, increased obsession with weight, or burn out and drop out.

The third component to consider when devising an exercise routine is regularity. Three to five times a week is considered regular. Aerobic kinds of exercise such as walking, biking, swimming, low-impact aerobics, hiking, rowing, and running offer the opportunity to engage in continuous physical activity in a moderate and regular way. You might also add light weight training, which strengthens your bones and skeletal muscles. Pick an activity you enjoy, since people rarely stick to exercise regimens that are too complicated, difficult, or boring. Plus, choose something you can do every day or every other day.

Don't overdo it by expecting too much of yourself. It makes it more likely that you'll give up on exercise completely. If you're not exercising at all currently, then start out slowly. For instance, if walking is of interest, take a walk around the block every other day for a week. Then increase the amount to two or three blocks the next week, and so on. Eventually, you'll increase the distance you go and the time you spend walking. Remember, moderate exercise means up to sixty minutes a day. You may want to contact your physician to make sure you have no health conditions that would prevent you from exercising.

If you're currently exercising too much (like two to three times a day or more than 60 minutes a day) then you need to cut back. Doing so may create an intense fear of gaining weight. Your body doesn't need that much exercise. Extreme amounts of exercise can strain your muscles, bones, heart, and lungs. Slowly decrease your amount of physical activity while also addressing any fears that arise (see chapters 3–7, "Game 1—Distorted Thinking: How to Refute Your Critic" and "Game 2—Perfectionism: End the Rejection Game," and "Affirm Yourself Daily: What You Say Can Heal You," chapter 3–8).

When you initially cut down your exercise, you might gain some weight. However, your weight will regulate itself over time, once your metabolism is allowed to function normally. If you're eating and exercising moderately and regularly, your body will weigh a healthy weight. You may want to consult a personal trainer or local gym to help you get started. Finding an exercise buddy can also help motivate you to be consistent and regular with your exercise.

Assignment: This is a great opportunity to set up your exercise routine. Use the *Weekly Exercise Chart* to make sure you're exercising enough and at a rate that builds muscle and burns fat. Develop a simple plan so you'll carry it through. Pick an activity you like and one that's convenient. Choose a time when you have the energy to do it. If you need to consult your physician before you begin, make that appointment.

WEEKLY EXERCISE CHART

List the kind of exercise, how many minutes you worked out, and your exercise pulse rate.

	FORM OF EXCERCISE	MINUTES	PULSE RATE
Day 1			
Day 2			
Day 3			
Day 4			
Day 5			
Day 6			
Day 7			

2 - 14

Stop Body Hate:
Accept Yourself Just the Way You Are

How long has it been since you liked the way your body looked, or you accepted your weight and size? The reason you keep starting new diets and/or exercise programs is to change your body so that it's acceptable to you. However, the results haven't lasted, so you search for a new diet or exercise regime with the hope of finally finding one that will permanently change your body into what you want it to be.

Even when you're able to change your body, it's never enough. You don't think you're thin enough or toned enough. After a diet, you gain the weight back, and sometimes even add more. Think about looking at pictures of yourself when you were either younger, thinner, or both. In hindsight, you look thin and attractive. Yet at the time, you probably didn't like your body or think it was thin enough. Now you wish you could go back to that body. This is a clear indication that your weight, size, and shape have not seemed satisfactory to you for a very long time, no matter what you've looked like.

Your body becomes an object of self-hatred. It is never enough: good enough, thin enough, toned enough, smooth enough, etc. Since all the regimens you have undertaken to this point have failed to work, why not try something else? What if you learned to accept your body the way it is today. Your first reaction is likely to be "No!"

"This is the only body you will ever have. You can keep neglecting, abusing, or 'whipping it into shape,' which hasn't seemed to work. Or, you can accept it as it is and start treating it well."

You know you'll never be able to pull that off. And if you do, then you're convinced you'll lose all motivation to lose weight. However, hating your body has not produced permanent weight loss. You have spent days, months, even years hating your body. How can you possibly have high self-esteem and a sense of self-worth with all that self-hatred going on?

Look at it this way. This is the only body you will ever have. You can keep neglecting, abusing, or "whipping it into shape," which hasn't seemed to work. Or, you can accept it as is and start treating it well. When you accept your body the way it is, you're much more likely to be gentle and kind to yourself.

Start by asking yourself to accept your body, not necessarily to love or even like it—that will come later. Accepting your body means accepting the reality of its size, shape, and weight; accepting exactly how it looks today—no judgments attached. It is what it is. Self-judgments don't allow any space for empathy or compassion. You create a win-win situation when you accept your body just the way it is. If you lose weight during the process of changing habits, great—you win. If you don't lose weight, or you lose less than you'd hoped to, then you still win because your body was okay in the first place.

The way to begin practicing body acceptance is to affirm that your body is okay today. Self-statements can be powerful in changing self-hatred to self-acceptance. The statement below conveys the message that your body is acceptable exactly the way it looks today.

Accepting Self-Statement: "Since I'm unwilling to take drastic measures to weigh what I want to weigh today, I accept myself as I am. I may change my mind tomorrow, but for today I accept myself exactly the way I am."

Give yourself the option of changing your mind the next day. However, for today, make the conscious commitment to say this statement to yourself. Counter every critical thought that pops into your head. When you say this to yourself every day, you'll probably notice a subtle difference within a few weeks. You'll begin to see that you're not only thinking less about your body, but the thoughts are less critical.

It may take months of continued reaffirmation to permanently change your old beliefs. You're bucking the narrowly defined cultural consensus of how every woman should look—rail thin. And men feel more pressure than ever before to be muscular and toned. But with this self-statement, your weight, shape, and appearance become less of an issue. You'll also develop a greater sense of accomplishment as your eating and exercise habits change to healthier, more balanced behaviors. This is because the focus is on changing behaviors first and seeing the weight loss as a permanent by-product of making those changes. This combination of changing habits and reducing critical thoughts will raise your self-esteem and sense of self-worth—something you've been striving for (consciously or unconsciously) for a very long time.

Adrianne is pear-shaped. Ever since the beginning of high school, she has tried to turn her body into a reed. For more than twenty years, she's used just about every diet and exercise program. None of them worked, and she felt more frustrated with each failed attempt. In fact, she found it harder to lose weight with each new diet, and no matter how much she exercised, she still had a small upper body compared to her waist and legs.

Adrianne consulted me when she began to realize that her genetic makeup was never going to change, and she was stuck in a diet mentality that seemed impossible to break. Once she let the reality of her genetics sink in, it took a while for her to accept the fact that she will never become long and lean. In addition to changing her eating and exercise habits, Adrianne and I discussed having her change her belief about her body instead of its shape. She had already proven to herself that changing the latter was impossible.

She began by really looking at herself in the mirror for the first time. She then challenged her belief that her body is unacceptable. She made self-statements that focused on accepting her body the way it was whenever critical thoughts about her body arose. Over the next few months as she continued to work on self-acceptance, she saw a positive difference in how she perceived herself. She became less critical of her body and liked that she doesn't have to feed it rabbit food or go to the gym for two hours every day. In fact, her body feels better since she has been eating and exercising more moderately. And she likes herself more than ever before.

Assignment: It's time to transform body hate into healthy self-acceptance. Use *Stop Body Hate* to list healthy self-statements you can make to counteract critical internal dialogues. You'll feel less depressed or anxious the more you accept the reality of your weight, shape, and appearance. It takes the pressure off while changing your eating and exercise habits because you aren't pushing yourself to look a certain way by a predetermined date. Give your body permission to take care of you and to adjust your weight naturally.

STOP BODY HATE

Accept the reality of how your body looks today—you don't have to love it yet, just own it. You have two choices: you accept it or you don't. Hating your body rarely motivates change. If it did, you would look the way you think you should by now.

Make a list of accepting self-statements about your body. Make sure the self-statements are nonjudgmental and factual. For instance, if you say to yourself, "My thighs are fat and I'm disgusted by them," you have labeled your legs as unacceptable. If you change that statement to, "My thighs are fine and I can live with them," you open the door to accepting your body.

ACCEPTING SELF-STATEMENTS ABOUT YOUR BODY

1. _____

2. _____

3. _____

4. _____

5. _____

6. _____

7. _____

8. _____

9. _____

10. _____

11. _____

12. _____

13. _____

14. _____

15. _____

16. _____

2 - 15

Face Your Feelings:
Alternatives to Feed Your Emotions

One of the main reasons people starve, binge, purge, or graze is to avoid facing painful or unpleasant emotions. When you choose to heal your physical self by changing your eating patterns and by exercising moderately, you will also need to learn to face your feelings instead of turning to food. Food, as I've said, has a numbing and soothing effect, so it's not always easy to change. But when you learn to experience your feelings without becoming overwhelmed, then you won't need food to soften the effect of your emotions.

"Feelings must be processed, not ignored."

Initially, many emotions may seem so powerful that you don't want to feel them. However, you can't resolve your feelings by denying they exist. And you can't hide them from yourself, either. Feelings must be processed, not ignored. That means first identifying them—trying to understand exactly what you are feeling and why—then actually feeling the emotion until the intensity decreases.

There are a number of ways to help yourself process feelings. Several are listed below. The goal is to feel your feelings from beginning to end. At first, you may only be able to tolerate an emotion for a few minutes before you find yourself turning to food for relief. Over time, as you practice experiencing your emotions, it will become easier to wait through the feelings and reach the other side, where the emotional intensity begins to decrease.

The only way you know you're really alive is through feelings—the pleasurable and the painful. Imagine a world with only intellect and no heart. It would be an empty place. When you can feel your emotions and experience them in your body, you are alive and connected to the world and to other people. You'll also get to know who you are and, thus, to develop and define a strong sense of yourself. The following techniques will aid you in experiencing and processing your feelings.

1. Sit Through Feelings: To prevent bingeing, grazing, purging, or starving, you must identify, experience, and sometimes act upon your feelings. This means feeling emotions instead of avoiding or denying them. Consider what is creating the feelings and notice how strong they are. Start with just five minutes of feeling the emotions. Feel them to their fullest intensity, which will move you through the experience and release the emotions—this is what processing means. Then you may need to devise ways to handle the situation or person who is stirring up the uncomfortable feelings. If a person or situation needs to be addressed, make a plan for what you're going to say or do. Sometimes you will deal directly with a person. At other times, you can experience your feelings on your own, then let them go.

When you decide to express your feelings to someone, make sure one of your goals is to resolve the situation and advance the relationship. Blowing off steam when you feel angry may give you momentary relief, but will it help you accomplish your aim—to change something in the way you and the other person interact? Your intent should not be to change the other person, but to attend to your own emotional self by acknowledging your feelings and then taking appropriate actions to help resolve them.

2. Write in a Journal: Keep a daily journal to assess which feelings and circumstances affect your eating behaviors. By keeping a "feelings journal," you can learn to identify, understand, and cope with your emotions. The very act of writing can bring tremendous relief, like a pressure cooker releasing steam. Write in the journal as if you're telling a friend what has happened to create the feelings. Once you understand and have experienced your feelings, you can make decisions about how to handle the event that caused these feelings.

"A strong support network helps decrease your sense of isolation, which comes from being secretive about eating behaviors."

As I mentioned, you may choose to deal with the situation or person, or to continue to process the feelings on your own. It's important to consistently write about your experiences so that you can become aware of patterns and progress. It's not so important to reread the journal, which can stir up unnecessary pain or embarrassment.

3. Call People: Cultivate supportive friends who understand what you're dealing with and who will gladly talk to you when difficult situations arise. A strong support network helps decrease your sense of isolation, which comes from being secretive about eating behaviors. You may have a group of people you call to discuss your feelings with and who share common life experiences. These may not be the people you talk to about food issues. Other friends may be the ones you call when you need to work through specific problems with food.

It's difficult and sometimes uncomfortable to confide in people who don't have the same struggles with food that you have. Therefore, joining a group and making connections with people who are dealing with the same issues can offer great support. When sharing feelings with friends, you feel supported at the time you're processing emotions. This can help you to build trust in others. It's important to learn who you can trust with your emotional experiences and who you can't. Pick people who are trustworthy and who will keep your confidence.

4. Pamper Yourself: Another main stimulus for bingeing, grazing, purging, or starving is the desire to soothe and calm yourself. Find other ways to create a sense of calmness—maybe bubble baths, long walks, massages, manicures, pedicures, meditation, or listening to music. Often, things that soothed you as a child will still soothe you as an adult. That's why so many people choose food.

Learn to choose other activities to take the place of food. You may not know what else calms you, or you may believe there is no time for frivolous activities. Consider then how much time you dedicate to eating behaviors, beginning with the thoughts and ending with the behaviors. If you spent that time pampering yourself instead, imagine all the ways you could give to yourself in a positive manner.

Pick an activity that feels good and do it instead of engaging in unhealthy eating behaviors. Start with one activity a week, then increase it to two activities a week, and so on. Don't overwhelm yourself with too much change so that you revert back to old behaviors. Just move at a pace that's manageable. If you do revert, get back on track the very next minute, next hour, or next day.

5. Exercise Moderately: Exercising in moderation can release tension. It also creates a physical sensation of feeling good. A variety of chemical reactions affect the body and help reduce stress and tension, elevate your mood, and create a sense of euphoria. Use "Get Moving! Exercise Will Change Your Weight the Easy Way" (chapter 2-13), as a guide for creating a balanced exercise program.

6. Calculate How Much Binges Cost: You'll be surprised to see how much money and time you spend on food. The next time you purchase binge or graze food, count both of the costs—how much money you spent and how much time you wasted in planning, buying, and eating the food. To calculate how much binge food costs you each year, use one binge-buying episode as an average cost per binge. Multiply this number by the amount of days you binge a month. Then multiply the result by twelve for all the months in the year. This will give you a rough estimate of how much money you spend in one year. You can do the same calculation to figure how much time you spend thinking about, planning, and then engaging in grazing, bingeing, or purging.

Imagine all the things you could buy, or how much money you could save if you didn't binge or graze. Think of what you could do with your time. Don't use this information to criticize yourself, use it to become informed and aware. This awareness can help you cut back on the number of binges you have.

7. Isolate Eating Behaviors: Right after bingeing, grazing, purging, or starving, consider the behaviors completed. Start over right then! Don't wait until tomorrow or next week to change behaviors. Every moment can be a new beginning.

It's too easy to say tomorrow will be different, so today anything is permissible. This is usually followed by a statement implying you will never do these behaviors again after the free-for-all of today. This kind of final statement can be too frightening and overwhelming. So begin now and go moment by moment or day by day instead of convincing yourself you will never do it again. As time passes, you'll notice that you have more days than not when you're engaging in healthy eating behaviors. When you go back to the old behaviors, getting back on track right away reduces the chance of self-punishment for "messing up." Everyone slips up and makes mistakes, including you. Go on from there.

"All weighing does is provide ammunition for self-criticism."

---

8. Stop Weighing Yourself: Most people can estimate their weight by how their clothes fit. They know immediately if they have gained or lost weight. Goal weights are often an arbitrary number chosen for various reasons: you weighed that in high school, that's what models weigh, the number sounds good, or your bones would stick out at that weight. However, that weight may be unachievable. Anorexics can attest to that. Thin is never thin enough. When your body doesn't weigh what you think it should, weighing yourself is a constant reminder of how you're failing. Continually weighing in keeps the focus on weight, shape, and appearance. Getting on the scale only serves as a momentary motivator to change. It doesn't last. If it did, you would have achieved the weight you wanted a long time ago. All weighing does is provide ammunition for self-criticism. When you stop constantly weighing yourself, your obsessive thoughts about weight will decrease, which will reduce the emphasis on your body. Wean yourself from using the scale. If you weigh yourself every day, go to every other day, then twice a week, then once a week, then once a month. Eventually, you'll reach a point where you can get on the scale only once or twice a year.

9. Get Rid of Benchmark Clothing: Give away or store all clothes that are too small. Keeping these clothes in the closet and periodically trying them on allows you to dwell on the perceived failure of your weight loss. Benchmark clothes become another scale to measure weight, size, and shape. When you give up weighing yourself, also get rid of benchmark clothing. Buy and wear clothes that fit comfortably. Smaller sizes rarely motivate permanent weight loss. It's just one more way to beat yourself up. Over time you can develop a level of comfort with the size of clothing that currently fits you.

10. Plan Activities: Get out of the house and try a new activity or participate in something you've been wanting to do for a while. Choose a positive alternative to unhealthy eating behaviors. Engaging in enjoyable activities decreases the likelihood that you'll turn to food because being good to yourself is incompatible with harming your body and your health.

When you're obsessed with food, buying items to eat can become a form of entertainment. However, once you begin eating meals on a regular basis, buying food evolves into a routine, not entertainment. Focusing on other activities will also become a habit. Pick activities you're interested in, that you have the time and money to pursue, and that are convenient. The easier and more interesting the activity, the more likely you are to stay involved with it.

Planning activities can include any number of things. Here are just a few ideas to get you thinking:

- Find a new hobby

- Join a group with a specific cause

- Learn a new sport

- Take up art, crafts, or needlework

- Take a class

- Volunteer

- Travel

- Explore local areas

- Start gardening

- Start a new business on the side

The list is endless and limited only by your imagination. Look around until you discover what interests you; then take a step each day until you're fully involved in the new activity.

11. Join a Group: There are two kinds of groups that help with food issues. One is run by a licensed therapist who is an expert in weight-management problems and/or eating disorders. Local hospitals or city and state psychological associations can help you get in contact with groups in your area. For more information, you can call the American Psychological Association (APA). The other kind of groups are offered through self-help organizations such as National Association of Anorexia Nervosa and Associated Disorders (ANAD), American Anorexia/Bulimia Association (AA/BA), Anorexia Nervosa and Related Eating Disorders (ANRED), National Eating Disorders Organization (NEDO), Overeaters Anonymous (OA), and Rational Recovery Systems (RRS). You can find these groups in your telephone book or in the References section in the back of this workbook.*

> *As Beverly began to change her eating behaviors, she found that there were periods in which her emotions seemed like they were on a roller coaster ride. There were also times of incredible calm. She hadn't been able to feel a range of emotions for years. She stifled both ends of the spectrum. Feelings she hadn't allowed herself to experience fully surfaced with surprising clarity and intensity. Beverly realized all that she had been covering up and not allowing herself to experience. The pleasurable feelings were much easier to handle, it was the painful ones that she wasn't sure she could deal with.*
>
> *She looked at her newly found feelings as an opportunity to get to know herself and see just what made her tick, emotionally. Instead of running to food every time she felt uncomfortable with her emotional life, she experimented with ways to be respectful of her emotional experiences. She first learned to identify what she was feeling and then to sit with it. In the beginning that wasn't easy. But it became easier with each attempt. She created a personal list of alternatives and used them to fill up her "coping bag." Every time she needed to deal with her feelings, she would decide the best way to do that. She became quite adept at dealing with her emotions instead of turning to food.*

12. Record Alternatives: Keep a daily record of the alternatives you used instead of engaging in unhealthy eating behaviors. You can use the chart on the following page for this.

Assignment: Use the *Alternatives Chart* to help you choose healthier options to starving yourself, bingeing on large amounts of food, purging to prevent weight gain, or grazing throughout the day. Pick three alternatives you can do on a regular basis. Once you use these consistently, select other ones you want to try. As you change your style of eating and exercise, more emotions will surface—so keep the list handy. The more you use these alternatives, the less you'll turn to food.

---

* Deirdra Price, Ph.D. does not endorse any organization listed on this page.

ALTERNATIVES CHART

Make a list of what you ate and whether you engaged in starving, bingeing, purging, or grazing. Then, list the situations, thoughts, or feelings that compelled you to use those behaviors and the alternatives you took instead.

Meal	Starve (x)	Binge (x)	Purge (x)	Graze (x)	Situation/ Thoughts/Feelings	Alternatives
Breakfast						
Snack						
Lunch						
Snack						
Dinner						

2 - 16

Relapse:
A Natural Stage of Healing

Changing your eating behaviors is never a perfect process. Most people have experienced a relapse at one time or another when they've tried to make changes. But relapses need not be permanent. Consider them just one of the many stages of healing. The first step in getting back on track is to understand the reasons you regressed to the old familiar behaviors. Being aware of the most common reasons will help you make choices once you've relapsed, so that the next time a relapse occurs you won't be caught off guard and will be able to pull yourself out of it more quickly. As time goes by, your new behaviors will become stronger, and you'll use healthier ways of coping with daily stresses and emotions. Eventually you'll avoid relapses altogether.

---

*"Weight gain is one of the most common reasons
for returning to eating-disordered behaviors."*

---

1. Weight Gain: This is one of the most common reasons for returning to eating-disordered behaviors. As you work toward making your eating regular and moderate, you may gain some weight, especially if you've been restricting calories or were purging a great deal. The weight gain is temporary. Once your eating is consistent and balanced, the weight will come off and your body will weigh what it knows to be healthy. Exercise adds the extra incentive your body needs to reduce weight. The weight may not match the number you want to see on the scale or the particular size of clothing you think you should wear, especially if the size or weight you've been aiming for would require extreme measures to achieve. However, it will be a healthy weight and you can learn to accept it. See "Stop Body-Hate: Accept Yourself Just the Way You Are" (chapter 2-14) and "Affirm Yourself Daily: What You Say Can Heal You" (chapter 3-8).

2. Feelings: Unpleasant feelings and stressful life events are common reasons for returning to old familiar behaviors. Like many people, you probably use food to avoid uncomfortable emotions. So one of the most frightening aspects of the healing process is the thought of having to handle all your feelings, which can seem too daunting or painful to experience on a daily basis. Remember, you're just learning how to tolerate your feelings. The only way to deal with them is to experience and process them; otherwise, they hang around begging to be addressed.

Because emotions play such an important part in initiating and maintaining eating disordered behaviors, a large part of this workbook is devoted to helping you cope with feelings (see "Face Your Feelings: Alternatives to Feed Your Emotions," chapter 2-15, and "Part Three: Healing the Emotional Self and Mental Self"). Over time, your emotions will become manageable without your having to turn to food to cope.

3. Deprivation: When you don't give yourself what you want, you desire it more. It's like suggesting that someone not think about a piece of cake...they can't help but think about the cake. Food deprivation leads to wanting the very thing that's forbidden, which eventually leads to bingeing.

The easiest way to prevent deprivation is to allow forbidden foods into your meal plans. This means giving yourself permission to eat moderate portions of what you really desire during a meal. If you really want it, have it. You may feel guilty afterwards, but the feeling will pass. As time goes by, you'll find it easier to eat a variety of foods without feeling guilty.

"Be understanding and forgiving with yourself throughout this process."

---

4. Perfectionism: Part of the reason people diet, starve, or purge is they believe these behaviors will lead to permanent weight loss and physical perfection. The desire to be perfect is part of the mental process of people who engage in eating-disordered behaviors. Because it's such an important component of the eating-disordered personality, I will address it specifically in "Part Three: Healing the Emotional Self and Mental Self" in "Game 2—Perfectionism: End the Rejection Game." Just as you expect perfection with your body, you'll also expect it in the healing process. But wanting change to be smooth and easy sets you up for a relapse.

Techniques you discover through trial and error are most helpful in the recovery process. However, if you expect to do everything perfectly the first time around, then you don't give yourself the freedom to practice or experiment to see what truly works best for you. That's why this workbook offers a variety of suggestions and techniques.

Some will work for you, some won't. You must learn what are the most helpful, and you are the best judge of what is successful. Be understanding and forgiving with yourself throughout this process.

5. Danger Zones: Knowing which situations are more likely to lead to starving, bingeing, grazing, or purging will help you prevent these behaviors in the first place. When you eat regularly and cope with feelings and daily stresses, two of the biggest reasons for turning to food or denying yourself food are removed. Figure out what sets you off. Keep handy your list of situations that are likely to lead to these behaviors (see "Recognize Your Danger Zones: Options to Food Abuse," chapter 2-11). By avoiding the circumstances or learning how to deal with them better, the danger zones soon fail to be dangerous.

Assignment: Be alert to the reasons why you might relapse. You'll want to cut short a relapse period and eventually prevent one altogether. You do this by becoming aware of what leads to a relapse in order to stop yourself from falling into the old eating patterns.

WHERE YOU ARE NOW

By the end of **Part Two: Healing the Physical Self**, you'll have the foundation to change your eating and exercise patterns into a healthier lifestyle. If you desire, go back to the areas you want to refine. Check (✓) the areas you have completed.

_____ You've read about the addictive nature of food-related problems and understand how stressful events lead you to starve, binge, purge, or graze.

_____ You've learned why diets don't work and assessed your diet history. You've seen how often you've lost weight only to gain it back again, and sometimes even more.

_____ You're practicing how to eat three meals a day, with or without snacks.

_____ You're learning how to plan meals on a daily or weekly basis.

_____ You're experimenting with eating balanced meals and moderate portion sizes.

_____ You're facing your fears and feelings of ambivalence that have stopped you from making changes in the past.

_____ You're expanding your food choices, eating more variety than you ever thought possible.

_____ You're learning how to eat in restaurants or fast-food establishments without overdoing it, and you feel less threatened by eating out.

_____ You're beginning to distinguish between physical and emotional hunger. You eat when you're physically hungry and take care of your feelings when you're emotionally hungry.

_____ You're incorporating your "bad" foods into mealtimes and eating those foods moderately (one to two servings).

_____ You've looked at your eating rituals and how you think they've helped you. Now you're reducing them by developing healthier eating habits.

_____ You're delaying and sometimes preventing starving, bingeing, purging, or grazing.

_____ You've created a balanced exercise routine and have started to exercise on a consistent basis.

_____ You're building healthy self-acceptance by using accepting self-statements to counteract critical internal dialogue.

_____ You're using a variety of healthy alternatives to cope with your feelings instead of turning to harmful eating behaviors.

_____ You know what makes you relapse, have taken steps to reduce the length of time in a relapse, and can eventually prevent a relapse altogether.

_____ You're letting your body decide what it wants to weigh. So if you're losing weight—great! If you're not—that's okay too!

With all the information you've acquired and all the behavioral changes you've made, you're now ready to move on to **Part Three: Healing the Emotional Self and the Mental Self.**

PART THREE: HEALING THE EMOTIONAL SELF AND THE MENTAL SELF

3 - 1

From Here to There:
How Beliefs Affect Choices

Your emotional experiences and your thought processes are closely linked. Ingrained beliefs, attitudes, and assumptions fuel your feelings, which then produce thoughts that reinforce your beliefs. From this vantage point, you make decisions and choices. Here's how it works. First, an event occurs that sets your beliefs in motion and results in feelings about the event. Thoughts arise to make sense of your feelings and to support your beliefs. You then decide how to behave and what actions to take.

Ted hates checking the board outside his economics class for test scores. He's afraid he's "failed" the test, which he defines as missing even one question. He believes he must get perfect scores on all tests, or at least the highest score and in the upper 90s. He finally summons the courage to find out his grade. When he sees his score of 91 and that five students have scored higher, he experiences a number of gut-wrenching emotions. Ted feels greatly disappointed, disgusted, frustrated, and angry with himself. He sees himself as a "failure."

Wracking his brain to figure out the questions he missed, he criticizes himself for making a number of mistakes: not studying harder, not focusing on the right things, not being smart enough to take the class. One lone thought enters his mind—that he did well by getting a 91! But the critical thoughts overtake him. To soothe the incredible pain he feels, he decides to go to the corner store and buy a big bag of M&M's. Ted vows that with the next test, he's going to stay up all night to study if necessary, to get the highest score. In the meantime, he heads home to eat his candy and play computer games to numb out.

The diagram below shows the relationship of all these components to each other.

Beliefs and Attitudes → Feelings and Thoughts → Decisions and Choices. [1]

The *beliefs*, *attitudes*, and *assumptions* you hold are developed during childhood and adolescence, and stored in your subconscious. They are based on the messages you

---

[1] "The Secrets of Manifesting What You Want, Part 1" Lazaris tape, © 1986 Concept: Synergy and is used by permission.

received from your parents, other significant persons, and society, as well as experiences you encountered. Beliefs are the foundation for how you *feel* and *think* about yourself, other people, and the world in general. From these you make your *decisions* and *choices*.

"When your beliefs become more positive and neutral...you will make better choices."

Powerful and significant changes occur by addressing either end of the spectrum—beliefs and attitudes or decisions and choices. If a belief is changed, everything else in the chain is affected and ultimately you make very different choices. Because your belief has changed, so have your feelings and the corresponding thought processes. When your beliefs become more positive or neutral, and your feelings are less painful, then not only is your thinking less critical or distorted, but you will make better choices.

Had Ted believed that doing his best is good enough instead of believing he must be perfect, the whole chain of events would have been altered. He would have seen the score of 91 and felt pleased and satisfied. He would have thought his efforts paid off and that he had done well considering how hard this economics test had been. Ted would have then planned a mini-celebration by doing what he loves most—playing tennis. He would have gone home and called his best friend to set up a tennis game, giving himself a break from studying for the rest of the day.

Likewise, if you make healthier decisions, your beliefs will be altered to match the information you gained by seeing a new outcome. Your thoughts and feelings are changed in the process.

For example, had Ted decided to go home and sit with his feelings instead of eating over them, he would have given himself the opportunity to tolerate and experience his painful emotions without hating himself for having them. This then would create the space to hear and refute his critical voice and challenge his beliefs. By not bingeing and making it through his emotional experience, Ted would learn that he doesn't have to binge to cope with emotions—his feelings won't kill him. By refuting his self-critical thoughts, his belief of perfectionism is chipped away, and he can begin to see that a score of 91 is pretty good; he will no longer despise himself for not achieving 100 percent. When Ted can do this on a regular basis, his beliefs will change, the critical voice will dissipate, and he will feel like he is handling life much better.

> *"When you can see yourself as a complete person*
> *with strengths* and *flaws, then having flaws is*
> *less painful—it's just part of being human."*

People who struggle with food, weight, and body image hold a universal belief that they should be perfect—in their appearance, how they present themselves, what they say, how they feel, and what they do. They put a great deal of time and energy into fixing flaws because they hate those parts of themselves. In Part Three, you'll learn how to accept those parts of yourself that you've been rejecting, reducing the veneer of perfection. When your beliefs demand and expect you to be perfect, the natural response is to hate, and therefore disown and ignore what you consider undesirable aspects of yourself. When you can see yourself as a complete person with strengths *and* flaws, then having flaws is less painful—it's just part of being human. When you can do this, you will develop a more balanced and complete view of yourself, tolerating *all* of your traits and characteristics.

Healing occurs within the emotional self and the mental self when you change your beliefs, understand and tolerate your emotional reactions as they relate to your beliefs, address your distorted and critical thought processes, and make healthier choices.

While Part Two provided techniques and strategies to help you deal with behaviors and cope with emotions directly, Part Three will help you to identify your beliefs and attitudes, and the feelings and thoughts that stem from them. It will show you how you reject parts of yourself because of your beliefs, which causes a great deal of pain and emotional suffering.

Part Three offers ways to help you make changes at all levels. Sometimes it's important to deal directly with the emotions and look no further. At other times, you'll work on your thought processes by exploring how you distort information. And yet again, it may be important to make a healthier choice and to try to do something differently. Often, you'll find it incredibly helpful and necessary to look at the underlying beliefs that are creating painful experiences so you can begin to make changes at the deepest level. Beliefs and attitudes are very powerful. They affect your viewpoint on just about everything, playing an important role in your everyday life.

In Part Three, you'll deal with your feelings and thoughts simultaneously, because they work in a synergistic fashion. You'll have an opportunity to identify your belief system, emotional reactions and thought processes, and what characteristics you disown. You'll also learn how to change the things that no longer work for you.

Assignment: Assess how your negative belief system affects the attitudes you hold, the feelings you experience, the thoughts you have, and the choices you make.

3 - 2

Understanding Your Crutch: Why You Use Food

The relationship between eating behaviors and emotions is complex. Certain feelings may seem too painful to bear, so, as a way of coping with the discomfort, you resort to

---

"When you were a child, you learned that food could offer support when life became unpleasant."

---

bingeing or grazing on food or starving yourself. As a child, you might not have been taught how to experience your emotions with comfort and ease. Instead, family members might have given you food to appease or calm you, or you discovered food for its soothing effect all on your own. When you were a child, you learned that food could offer support when life became unpleasant. That's why you choose food over other substances, such as alcohol or drugs (although people who turn to food may also use other substances for similar reasons). The way your parents, extended family, close friends, and even teachers approached food has had a great influence on you.

Food may have been used to:

1. Console you when you felt upset. Parents or grandparents may have given you food to comfort you. As an adult, you may be able to recall those "comfort foods" that reduced your level of distress.

2. Quiet you. Parents bank on food for its ability to "anesthetize" or temporarily calm their child's emotions. This formula worked from day one when, as an infant, you cried for milk and were quieted once you were fed.

3. Distract you from feelings your parents were uncomfortable seeing you display—often a reflection of emotions parents aren't able to tolerate within

themselves. A child can become so wrapped up in eating that he or she stops crying, screaming, yelling, pouting, fussing, or fidgeting.

4. Help you cope with life's stresses. People who struggle with their weight and food often have parents who modeled turning to food to handle life's ups and downs. The parents also used food to calm down, numb out, or feel nurtured.

5. Reward or punish you. You may have been given something to eat when you were "good," and food may have been denied when you were "bad."

"How parents feel about food is conveyed to their children."

---

6. Serve as an instrument of power and control. When you didn't follow your parents' guidance, food may have been withheld or pushed on you. This kind of behavior is often used at the dinner table when the whole family sits down together. A common example is when a parent makes the child sit at the table until everything on the plate is finished—and the child sits there until midnight.

How parents feel about food is conveyed to their children. If parents have issues with food, the child senses it and is more likely to become wary of food as well. The classic example is the parent who continually diets and passes on the belief that certain foods are "dangerous" and therefore forbidden. The child then grows up with poor eating habits and a diet mentality of weight management.

When a parent expresses dissatisfaction with his or her body, it's more likely that a child will learn to dislike his or her body. This is reinforced when the parent comments on the child's inadequate body parts. The child then develops body hate and later, as an adult, may take drastic and extreme measures to alter her or his appearance.

Because of what's modeled in the home, people who engage in unhealthy eating behaviors believe they shouldn't have unpleasant feelings. When they do experience painful emotions, they feel out of control, as if their emotional self has a life of its own—somewhat like an alien force. Your emotions aren't alien, however, they're very much a part of you. Because painful emotions can be so disconcerting and destabilizing, you disown and label them as unacceptable. And you turn to food to deal with them.

Your beliefs and attitudes concerning events and circumstances in your life will stir up feelings. This affects your decisions about how you're going to cope with feelings. How you cope is often modeled after how your parents did. So it's important to recognize why you choose or deny yourself food to avoid experiencing these feelings. When you understand the reasons you turn to food, you've taken the first step on the path to owning, accepting, and dealing with your emotions.

Below is a list of the most common reasons why people turn to food, starve themselves, or purge. Check (✓) the ones that apply to you. If you check two or more of the statements, you have a problem with using food to cope with your emotions.

Do you use food:

_____ When you feel physically hungry or deprived of certain kinds of foods?

_____ To stifle or numb your feelings?

_____ To comfort or nurture yourself, or to feel taken care of?

_____ To calm down or create a sense of relaxation?

_____ To distract yourself and avoid difficult issues by escaping from reality?

_____ To feel in control when life feels beyond your control?

_____ To momentarily fill an internal emptiness?

_____ To procrastinate attending to responsibilities?

_____ To alleviate boredom?

_____ To feel energized?

_____ As a punishment for being bad?

_____ As a reward for being good?

Assignment: Once you've identified the reasons why you turn to food, fill out the *Food Use Chart*. You'll be able to assess what feelings you're avoiding or reinforcing when you reach for, push away, or purge food.

FOOD USE CHART

List why you use food and what you're avoiding or reinforcing. For example, when you use food as punishment, you're reinforcing your belief in how bad you are. And when you use food to numb your feelings, you're avoiding dealing with them.

FOOD'S USE	AVOIDANCE/REINFORCEMENT
1.	
2.	
3.	
4.	
5.	
6.	
7.	
8.	
9.	
10.	
11.	
12.	
13.	
14.	
15.	
16.	
17.	
18.	

3 - 3

The Power of Negative Beliefs:
How History Shaped You

You are who you believe you are. If you have positive beliefs about yourself, you're more likely to interpret experiences as positive and to maintain self-esteem when unpleasant situations occur. In general, you'll feel good about who you are and you'll like yourself. Conversely, if you have negative beliefs about yourself, you're more likely to interpret life's experiences as painful, frustrating, or unsatisfying; to dislike yourself; to feel depressed and/or anxious; and to blame yourself for any perceived failures. Just as you do with yourself, you also hold a variety of beliefs about other people, and your beliefs shape how you feel about, think, and react to those individuals.

"We all form our beliefs in childhood and adolescence."

The positive beliefs you have about yourself create self-esteem and self-worth. Don't change these. The negative beliefs are the ones that hamper your personal sense of value and importance. These are the ones that will be addressed in Part Three.

We all form our beliefs in childhood and adolescence. We get spoken and unspoken messages from adults that tell us who we are, how we look, how well we perform, and how we should feel and think. These messages affect a child's and adolescent's sense-of-self, self-esteem, and self-worth. Most of this information comes from parents and other significant persons.

Women who have bulimia consistently describe growing up in families with similar kinds of dynamics. They characterize their families as less encouraging of assertive or self-sufficient behaviors. They also view their families as having experienced a great deal of conflict, though they were discouraged from openly and directly expressing their feelings to other family members.

Negative, critical messages like these produce young people who lose their ability to create a positive self-image. A sense of not being good enough emerges. As they grow up, they learn to reject the flawed aspects of themselves because their parents found those characteristics unacceptable. They begin to strive for perfection, hoping to please their parents and aching to feel good about themselves. It doesn't work. Their attempts are doomed to failure because their foundation for a positive sense-of-self has been weakened, and they're unable to see themselves in a positive light.

"No matter what messages a child or adolescent receives while growing up, they believe them to be true."

Children raised in this sort of environment are more likely to develop a negative belief system about themselves. No matter what messages a child or adolescent receives while growing up, they believe them to be true. So when the feedback is harsh and critical, that's what they believe. Most often, it's not facts that adults are passing on to their child but the adults' own negative *beliefs* about the child. Children, however, assume they're facts, since they're unable to tell the difference between facts and beliefs.

A number of things happen as a result of the negative and critical messages children receive during childhood and adolescence:

1. They develop their own negative beliefs and attitudes, which eventually affect the way they perceive reality.

2. Those negative beliefs produce painful feelings about the self.

3. They have corresponding thought processes that make sense of the feelings, and they play "mind games" to reinforce the negative belief system.

4. Different parts of the self develop, each part participating in playing the games.

5. How they interpret an event has a direct effect on the decisions and choices they then make. For example, over time, their body becomes the path for experiencing control when other aspects of life feel beyond control. When they can't stop unpleasant feelings or critical thoughts, they choose food to numb out, to create a sense of comfort, and to reduce tension within their bodies. The body's outer appearance is controlled by forcing it to fit the familial or societal ideal (beliefs) through extreme measures, such as restrictive dieting, overexercising, diet pills, or drugs and various forms of purging (choices).

> *Harold believes he's fat. His grandparents and aunt on his father's side always told him so. Every summer, when he visited them, they would comment on his body and what he ate—alluding that his "baby fat" had to go. Harold learned to dislike his body and feels disgusted with it most of*

the time. He tells himself, in quite critical terms, how gross his body is and that no one will love him when he looks this way. Objectively, Harold's weight is within the normal range. Yet, he continually diets with the hope of molding himself, through his body, into someone lovable. It hasn't happened yet. As a matter of fact, as time goes by, he likes himself less and less, and diets more and more.

All of the internal players—the negative beliefs and attitudes the person holds, and the corresponding feelings and thought processes (i.e., the games played)—are described in Part Three. Once negative beliefs are changed and distorted thought processes are altered, then feelings about and perceptions of the self are much more realistic and balanced. The decisions you make are then much more likely to be constructive, not destructive.

"Information gives you power. When you know what's happening and can see what you're doing and why, then you can begin to make changes."

Part Three can be difficult and intense at times. You may want to consider seeking support from a therapist or friend while working through it, since it can stir up feelings you might have normally avoided by engaging in harmful eating behaviors. Once you start practicing healthier eating behaviors, many feelings will become stronger because you're no longer using food to mask their intensity. Other feelings will decrease in magnitude and even fade away.

Information gives you power. When you know what's happening and can see what you're doing and why, then you can begin to make changes. If you unconsciously do the same thing over and over again and don't know why, then there's no opportunity to change. Being conscious of your belief system, feelings, thoughts, and decisions gives you the option to do things differently. You have many more choices than you ever thought you had. It's up to you as to how much support you need while healing the emotional self and the mental self.

Assignment: Explore how your negative belief system developed and how your beliefs influence your feelings and thoughts about yourself, other people, and life events. See how you make choices on a daily basis because of what you believe. Make the link between negative beliefs and your focus on weight and appearance.

3 - 4

Your Players:
The Critic, Child, Adolescent, and Healer

The self is made up of different parts. When you received negative messages during childhood and adolescence, certain parts of yourself believed those messages. You had little choice, and therefore bought into the prevailing belief system. As an adult, certain parts of the self play a role in reinforcing negative beliefs and attitudes. Once you identify these internal players and understand the games they play, you can learn to change the negative beliefs and distorted thought processes, and stop playing the games. Doing so will positively affect how you feel about and see yourself.

The Critic

This part of the self enforces internal rules based on the belief system developed during childhood and adolescence. The dialogue many people hear in their heads is a barrage of critical comments that ensure that feelings, thoughts, and behaviors (decisions) stay in line with the negative beliefs. These self-statements are automatic and conditioned. Your critic knows no other belief system, only the one taught by the adults who had an impact on you while you were growing up.

The critic's reinforcement of beliefs serves many purposes. Ultimately, the critic offers protection. It makes sure that you don't fully trust other people, which guards you against being hurt or betrayed. To guarantee you'll get approval from others, the critic pushes you to engage in efficient, helpful, people-pleasing behaviors. The downside to having a critic is that it doesn't allow the development of self-trust or self-esteem.

---

*"If you listen to what your critic says, it sounds
similar to what you heard while growing up."*

It second guesses any decision you make based on intuition, using instead your negative belief system as a guide. The critic does the very same thing parents and other important adults did. It's no different because the critic patterns its comments after the messages you received while growing up and does not deviate from them. If you listen to what your critic says, it sounds similar to what you heard while growing up. You may even be able to discern whose voice and belief system the critic patterns itself after.

To become familiar with your critic, listen to the critical comments inside your head: "I'm fat." "I'm ugly." "I never do things right." "I'm unlovable." These self-statements seem like they're facts; they're not. They're beliefs, and beliefs can be changed. However, the critic doesn't want this to happen because it was created specifically to enforce negative beliefs. This is how you've maintained your loyalty to your parents or other significant persons. When you introduce new beliefs that don't match or are the opposite of the original set of negative beliefs, the critic will refute them and repeat the old beliefs more loudly. Whenever you attempt change, the critic will put up a fight. It knows no other way, and all other options seem inferior. This doesn't mean you cannot make changes, you can. You needn't get rid of your critic, just learn how to work with it. The critic's main mode of operation is playing mind games. The first step toward getting to know your critic is to understand the games it plays. Then you can make changes from there.

The critic is closely related to three other parts of the self—the child, the adolescent, and the internal healer. There are other parts that delineate the self, however, the parts mentioned in this chapter are those mainly involved in reinforcing and keeping the negative beliefs alive. The three parts are linked together and often work in tandem. The child and adolescent learned the beliefs, the critic reinforces them, and the healer is looking for ways to help you accept yourself and make the necessary changes to feel better about yourself.

The Child

Childhood brings both pleasurable and painful experiences. You cannot make it through childhood without being wounded; it's an inevitable part of growing up. Many parents and other significant persons don't mean to hurt a child. Their intention is to help the child grow into a responsible, conscientious adult. However, the way they go about it wounds the child. Some adults, however, intentionally want to hurt a child—which can make the wounding seem so much more profound and painful. When you look back on your childhood, you'll be able to tell the difference between intentional and unintentional woundings.

All wounding experiences have a similar theme. The adult gives the child negative and critical messages about how the child is inadequate in some way. The child clearly feels the adult's disappointment. Yet, no matter what the child does at that time to win favor, it's met with disapproval.

"For most people, one particular wounding
stands out as the most painful."

Some wounds are bigger than others. For most people, one particular wounding stands out as the most painful. It might be a parental divorce, cruel peer teasing, the death of a family member or friend, severe illness, a parent who strove for perfection and made sure the child did too, a parent who was hostile when the child made a mistake, physical or emotional abandonment, or emotional, physical, or sexual abuse. There can also be a pattern in which the child is regularly wounded, and many of these experiences carry the same theme. Because of this, there may be many times during a person's childhood that they were touched by these kinds of experiences.

> *Justine experienced a common kind of wounding, similar to other people who struggle with food. She was yelled at and admonished for expressing unpleasant feelings, especially if the feelings were directed toward her parents. When Justine expressed anger about something one of her parents did, her father got angry in return and punished her. He would say, "Don't talk like that. You're being disrespectful!" And he grounded her from playing with her best friend the next day. Justine felt ashamed for expressing her anger. Her father had a difficult time tolerating and accepting Justine's anger and, therefore, didn't teach her effective coping strategies. Her mother didn't intervene. She let her husband handle the disciplining. Justine's father repressed her expression of feelings, just as his parents had done to him.*
>
> *Justine learned that showing anger was unacceptable in her family. So when she experienced anger, she became upset with herself and disowned this aspect of her emotional self. She did this by becoming highly self-critical of her emotions just like her parents were. Justine learned to turn off her feelings—by eating all the cookies in the cookie jar. After that, she didn't feel so angry. As a matter of fact, she felt quite sedated.*

Shame is one of the major emotions a child feels when wounded[2]. Appropriate amounts of shame help a child to learn right from wrong, to feel remorse, to grow, and to change. However, when an adult uses extreme amounts of shame on a child, it becomes debilitating and destructive to the child for a number of reasons:

1. The child learns to feel guilty about every error or mistake made

---

[2] Much of the information on shame comes from "Ending Shame, Part I: Infancy," "Ending Shame, Part II: Psychic Contracts of Pain (Childhood)," "Ending Shame, Part III: Those Adolescent Years," and "Ending Shame, Part IV: Adult Shame" Lazaris tapes, © 1990 Concept: Synergy and is used by permission.

2. The child develops little, if any, trust in her or his ability to make decisions based on feelings, instinct, or gut reactions

3. Self-esteem is low due to near constant critical internal dialogue

4. Self-worth is minimal

Shame is passed from one person to another. When adults shame a child, they're passing on the shame they received as a child. But children don't realize they're taking on someone else's shame, fueled by that person's internalized belief system. Rather, children begin to believe there is something wrong with them and that they're being told about it. The child has no idea that negative beliefs are being passed on through the act of shaming. Statements adults make to a child during the wounding process build the foundation for negative beliefs and the critical internal dialogue that stems from the beliefs. Statements that form negative beliefs sound like: "Stop eating that cake, or you're going to get fat." "No one will ever love you if you act like that." "Don't you cry!" "I'm putting you on this diet for your own good." "Once you lose weight, then you'll look pretty." "We'll go clothes shopping when you lose five pounds." "You can't have cake like your sister can, she's thin." "Either you get an 'A' on your math test, or you're grounded." "You look fat in that outfit." "Don't talk back to your mother like that."

"Shame is easier to feel than pain."

This is when a child begins to reject the parts of him/herself seen as undesirable. If the adults around them think aspects of the child are not acceptable, the child will think the same. The flaws are the very things the critic criticizes.

Underneath the shame is the actual pain felt during the wounding experience. Shame is much easier to feel than pain. The pain gets buried and shame is readily felt throughout life. As these children grow into adulthood, they're likely to pass on their unresolved shame to their children, partners, other family members, friends, coworkers, and acquaintances by creating similar wounding experiences for these people.

The child (or children of different ages, depending on how many wounding experiences there were) holds the memories and emotions attached to these experiences. As long as the child continues to see the world through the beliefs formed during these experiences, the critic has the power to reinforce negative beliefs about the self. They work in tandem: the child learns the beliefs and the critic reinforces them. Once the child in you can release the pain, change beliefs, stop the self-shaming, and accept flaws, the critical internal dialogue will decrease because your critic no longer has the list of negative beliefs from which to operate. Positive and neutral beliefs will have replaced the old ones, and these new beliefs will be reinforced.

To accomplish this, you must first become familiar with your inner child. One of the best ways to start the process is by looking at pictures taken of you when you were a child. Reminisce about your childhood. See what images and memories come to mind. See if you can recall what you looked like, what you wore, how your hair was fixed, and what you were doing. Does a certain age come to mind? Why that age? For some people it takes a while to access the child that was wounded and shamed; for others it's quite easy. There may be many ages that come to mind. Some parts of you may feel wounded, other parts are free from those kinds of painful experiences. Notice what experiences and memories come up; they are significant.

Once the child has your attention, she or he will begin to communicate with you if given the opportunity. The child has always said things to you, although it may have been difficult to distinguish that voice from everything else you say to yourself. The child may be demanding or shy. Pay attention to the themes of statements made or requests for needs being met. Most likely, the messages center around negative information received during childhood or deficits where basic needs weren't met. The wounded child is stuck in the mindset of the wounding experiences where the negative beliefs were formed. The child can be helped, and the first step is getting to know the child and the experiences that created the shame and pain.

The Adolescent

Adolescence is a time of great change, confusion, and excitement. A wide variety of events and experiences happen during this period, as young people explore and solidify their senses of identity. Some experiences are wonderful; others wind up wounding the adolescent.

Everyone goes through a time in adolescence when they feel invincible, as if nothing could destroy them. It's that indestructibility that causes adolescents to take more risks and be more adventurous than adults. Yet something happens to adolescents that shatters that sense of invincibility. Within adolescence, as in childhood, there may be a pattern of being wounded. Still, one experience is likely to stand out as the one that altered everything and led to a loss of faith in and distrust of themselves and perhaps others. Adolescent woundings often center around themes of physical changes, sexual development, independence, privacy, and relationships with newly developing love interests. From this point on, the adolescent no longer feels invincible. Other feelings predominate instead, like insecurity, hesitancy, wariness, guardedness, distrust, depression, anxiety, and hurt.

Alan remembers the incident that changed his whole outlook on life. He was feeling pretty confident in the tenth grade, but also a bit sensitive and shy. When he earned a spot on the junior varsity basketball team, he saw it as an opportunity to meet girls and hang out with the cool crowd. He'd been keeping a journal of his deepest thoughts and feelings, carrying it wherever he went so he could jot down what he was thinking or feeling at any moment in time. One day after basketball practice, when he was changing back into his school clothes, he realized someone had broken into his locker and taken the notebook containing his writings. The next day, photocopied pages from the journal were taped on the locker room schedule board. Alan was mortified when his peers laughed and pointed at him. He took down all the copies he could find and tore them up, vowing to never write about his thoughts or feelings again. He beat himself up for writing such stupid, sensitive things. He became depressed for weeks.

Alan never found out who stole his writings, but from that day on, he buried his emotional self so deep that he was unable to clearly recognize or acknowledge what he felt or how his emotions affected him. He didn't trust his emotions, nor did he trust others. Both could betray him.

Whenever Alan's feelings became too strong, he would stop eating. He discovered that he gained a fleeting sense of emotional control from using this tactic whenever necessary to avoid experiencing or displaying his emotional side. He has been using starvation for years to ward off his feelings and gain a sense of control. Once his feelings subside, he resumes eating. Starving doesn't work as well for him as it did in the beginning. He keeps doing it because he knows of no other way to cope with his feelings, and expressing them seems too dangerous.

As you look back and explore your own adolescence, many experiences may come to mind. However, one specific experience created a loss of faith in yourself. From that point on, your adolescent intuition and inner knowing became buried. How could you, the adolescent, believe in instincts and emotions when you no longer trusted yourself?

During adolescence, the critic gains more power because the original beliefs learned in childhood become more solidified and entrenched. The critic then plays mind games based on the belief system. Listening to the intellect and beliefs becomes safer and more predictable than relying upon and trusting any intuitive sense of knowing.

Had Alan been able to see that having his notebook stolen was part of an adolescent prank and not an assault on his character, he may have been able to bounce back and continue his writings—but not carry his notebook with him. This was an opportunity to express more fully what he thought and felt because the incident certainly stirred up many reactions. Instead, he decided to shut down, solidifying his belief that his feelings were "unmanly." Whenever he felt something he deemed unacceptable, he severely criticized himself for doing so, which turned off his emotions. He employed starvation to seal the emotional coffin so none of his feelings would escape.

During adolescence, the process of deciding what is acceptable and unacceptable about the self continues. The adolescent rejects and casts off those parts of the self deemed unacceptable. These flaws are seen as the enemy. Childhood desires for attaining perfection beckon more strongly in adolescence as the promised path to happiness and self-liking. Because perfection is an unattainable ideal, however, the adolescent always ends up frustrated and disappointed for not measuring up. Yet, since flaws are intolerable, a pattern of striving for that illusive perfection begins to predominate in everything undertaken. The goal is to become perfect, rather than to know and tolerate the complexity and richness of the full self.

The process of recognizing the adolescent is much the same as recognizing the child. See what images and experiences come to mind. Does an age jump out at you? What happened at that age to take away your sense of invincibility and confidence? What parts of the self do you see being rejected?

"Every one of us has a healer within who believes we're okay just the way we are."

Your adolescent may be hiding; listen for that young adult voice. The messages, needs, and desires sound different than the child's—they're more mature. Much like the child, though, the adolescent reiterates self-statements reflecting negative beliefs, because the wounding experience during this time of development confirmed those beliefs. Once you understand the wounding experience, you can take steps toward healing the pain and shame that led to distrusting yourself and others.

The Healer

Every one of us has a healer within who believes we're okay just the way we are. The healer doesn't expect perfection. Instead, the healer continually guides us in our development of self-acceptance and a sense of self-love, in listening to the whispers of intuition and wisdom, and in fostering nonjudgmental compassion. But we cannot hear the healer clearly with the critic loudly and consistently reinforcing negative beliefs.

When you address your childhood and adolescent woundings, and the critical voice gets softer, then the healer becomes easier to hear. Old beliefs no longer cloud the gentle voice of the healer. The difficulty comes in knowing how to access it. You can hear the healer when you think about engaging in destructive or unhealthy eating behaviors. You'll notice a second thought counters those thoughts, telling you to not engage in the behaviors. You also access the healer when you consciously offer yourself compassion and understanding for what you're going through. The healer provides constant acceptance when you allow yourself to suspend judgments of self and others. Listen beyond the critical messages. A subtle thought will bubble up. This is the healer offering helpful guidance.

To recognize the healer, listen to the message of the healthy things you want to say to and do for yourself. The healer gives many suggestions and words of encouragement. This voice often says something like: "I can deal with my feelings and not binge." "I can let this food digest in my body." "I don't have to throw this up." "I am a good person." "My weight is okay right now." "Even though these feelings are painful, they are part of me and I can live through them."

You may continue to opt for harmful eating behaviors and critical self-judgments for a while. However, the healing voice offers other options. The healer is compassionate and patient. Sometimes it takes listening closely, especially when working through negative beliefs and critical thinking. But with guidance from your internal healer, healthier choices will emerge. Begin to act on those choices as the healing process progresses.

Assignment: Meet the different parts of your self—the critic, child, adolescent, and healer. Identify how your critic, child, and adolescent play a role in maintaining your harmful eating habits and poor self-image. Explore how you were shamed and why this colors your view of yourself and the world in general. When you define your shame and pain, you can then begin the process of healing. Listen for the subtle voice of your healer, who can help you make positive changes.

3 - 5

You Are What You Believe: Your View of the World

Beliefs and attitudes are the driving force in how we perceive ourselves and the world. As our belief system becomes solidified and ingrained, the critic reinforces negative beliefs through harsh and critical self-statements. These self-statements lead to decisions about how we behave and how we let our beliefs guide our choices. This makes the beliefs seem very real.

> *"We automatically retain incoming information that supports and reinforces our beliefs, and discard all other information."*

For example, when you believe you're fat, feelings of self-disgust and hatred get stirred up. Your critic chimes in, calling you weak and lazy. You then decide to go on a crash diet to prove to yourself that you're not a slouch and you can lose weight. However, when the diet fails, you feel frustrated, depressed, and hopeless. Your critic makes sure you're aware of how fat you still are and how you can't get this dieting thing right. Eventually you jump on the dieting bandwagon again, with the hope of losing weight and finally feeling good about yourself. You're so busy going on and off diets that you don't consider that it's your belief that's causing the turmoil and needs to be changed—not necessarily your weight.

We automatically retain incoming information that supports and reinforces our beliefs, and discard all other information. Consequently, beliefs become rigid, unbending, and life-guiding. We blindly follow the belief as if it's etched in stone and cannot be erased.

Assignment: Fill out the checklist on the next pages to identify your personal set of negative beliefs. Once you understand what you believe, you can see how your beliefs color your perceptions and influence how you behave.

As you develop an awareness and understanding of your personal negative beliefs, it becomes easier to see how they get played out from situation to situation.

Check (✓) the beliefs and attitudes that apply to you.

1. I expect to have only positive and pleasant thoughts and feelings. _____

2. I want control over my emotions at all times. _____

3. I must be perfect or I am nothing. _____

4. When I reach perfection, I will be happy. _____

5. I can never make mistakes. _____

6. I must be good at everything I do. _____

7. I must please everyone all the time. _____

8. Everyone must like me. _____

9. Other people's needs are more important than mine. _____

10. Other people's opinions matter more than mine. _____

11. My parents are/were always right. _____

12. Everyone hates fat people. _____

13. I need to be thin to be happy. _____

14. When I get thin, I will be happy. _____

15. I will never be thin enough. _____

16. No one will want me or love me if I'm fat. _____

17. I must be thin at all costs. _____

18. The harder I work, the happier I will be. _____

19. No pain, no gain. _____

20. It's disgusting to be lazy or procrastinate. _____

21. I am a weak person. _____

22. I am ugly. _____

23. I am fat. _____

24. I'll never be where I want to be. _____

25. I have to be a certain way for others to love and accept me.   _____

26. My parents (or partner) expect a lot of me.   _____

27. My parents (or partner) want to control me.   _____

28. I can never do enough to please my parents (or partner).   _____

29. I don't deserve good things.   _____

30. Sometimes I believe I am a bad person.   _____

31. When I'm bad, I must be punished.   _____

List other beliefs and attitudes you hold that are different than the preceding ones.

1. _____

2. _____

3. _____

4. _____

5. _____

6. _____

7. _____

8. _____

9. _____

10. _____

11. _____

12. _____

13. _____

14. _____

15. _____

16. _____

3 - 6

How You Feel and Think: What Choices Are They Driving?

Your belief system guides your emotional reactions and thought processes. Negative beliefs often stir up powerful, uncomfortable, and overwhelming feelings that lead to distortions in your perception of reality. Your critic helps reinforce your perceptions,

---

"It can become depressing and anxiety producing to constantly think critical thoughts about yourself."

---

which are dictated by your beliefs. It can become depressing and anxiety producing to constantly think critical thoughts about yourself. Who wouldn't feel depressed or anxious with all that negative self-feedback? Many people put so much energy into unhealthy eating behaviors because those behaviors help to numb and stifle the effects of such intense emotional experiences. Once you develop an understanding of your emotional reactions and thought processes, it becomes easier to see their relationship to your belief system, and the choices you make because of them.

Assignment: Fill out the checklist below to help you understand your thought processes and emotional reactions. You'll see how your belief system influences what you feel and think and, ultimately, your decisions.

Check (✓) the thoughts and feelings that apply to you.

1. I feel guilty when I get angry or mad.   _____

2. I feel guilty and wrong for having negative feelings toward
   other people.   _____

3. I often get upset, scream, yell, or cry but can't say why.   _____

4. I think highly critical thoughts about myself.   _____

5. I have to be perfect to be okay. _____

6. I must be good at everything I do. _____

7. I always compare myself to other people. _____

8. I wonder what other people think of me. _____

9. I think other people are better than me. _____

10. I feel guilty when I have negative thoughts about my parents
    or other people. _____

11. I worry about what my parents or other people think of me. _____

12. I worry how people will react if I say "No" to them. _____

13. I find that in general, I worry a lot. _____

14. I feel depressed or blue much of the time. _____

15. At times, I feel anxious or panicked. _____

16. I take on too much responsibility. _____

17. I think I must do things for other people but not for myself. _____

18. I don't deserve good things. _____

19. I think I'm a greedy person. _____

20. I feel like a fake. _____

21. I feel guilty when I do something enjoyable, instead of working. _____

22. Everything I do seems routine and boring. _____

23. I want more direction in life. _____

24. I feel stuck and want to change, but I don't know what to change
    or how. _____

25. I'm afraid of change. _____

26. I'm afraid of making the wrong decision. _____

27. I feel paralyzed. _____

28. I hate to waste time. _____

29. I want to be alone much of the time. _____

30. I feel isolated and am afraid to be alone. _____

31. I constantly think about my body, weight, shape, and appearance. _____

32. I feel like I'm a bad person. _____

33. I feel like I need to be punished for being bad. _____

List other feelings and thoughts you hold that are not mentioned on the previous pages.

1. _____

2. _____

3. _____

4. _____

5. _____

6. _____

7. _____

8. _____

9. _____

10. _____

11. _____

12. _____

13. _____

14. _____

15. _____

16. _____

17. _____

18. _____

3 - 7

The Mind Games:
Stop Playing and Win

You have a set pattern for how you think about and interpret events occurring in your world. These patterns can be considered "mind games." Initially, they provided a way for you to mentally organize and understand your evolving belief system, helping you make sense of incoming information. Mind games then became ingrained ways of perceiving reality. They're consistent and predictable even though some create a negative self-evaluation that results in emotional distress. Eventually, you view each situation through the lenses of the mind games.

You play mind games quite unconsciously. At one time, you may have been consciously aware of what you were thinking and why, but now the reasons are lost, and the way you think happens quite automatically. Once these games become entrenched, you become sure your style of thinking and perceiving the world is accurate and unchangeable. Even when it's painful to see yourself and the world in the way you do, you cling to mind games.

When you can become conscious of your thought processes and are able to make changes in them, your perceptions of and feelings about yourself and others will change. As mentioned before, when you hold positive or neutral beliefs about yourself, you will have positive feelings and a more realistic and balanced view of yourself.

People who struggle with food, weight, and body image use similar mind games. Five different mind games are described on the following pages: Distorted Thinking, Perfectionism, Watchful Eye, Nonassertiveness, and Anticipation. They're written about as if they're separate, yet they interrelate and intertwine with one another.

Game 1
Distorted Thinking:
How to Refute Your Critic

Distortions in thinking are ingrained ways of perceiving reality. Everyone interprets reality using internal programming developed from repetitive messages received during childhood and adolescence. If children receive harsh and critical feedback about who they are, a negative belief system unfolds. This creates distortions in thinking that acts as a screen, allowing certain information in and excluding other information. Negative information that matches the beliefs is accepted as truth, and positive information that counters the beliefs is rejected as flattery. This way of perceiving reality eventually becomes rigid and automatic.

The critic in you uses distorted thinking to confirm that you're messing up—not measuring up—and being imperfect. This leads you to dislike yourself and you discount yourself based on your perceived flaws. You wind up feeling depressed or anxious because the barrage of self-criticism makes you focus on the flawed aspects of yourself. Depression is closely related to self-esteem—when you feel depressed, you experience low self-esteem. And your self-esteem and self-worth are intimately connected to how you perceive yourself. So, over time, when you continually criticize yourself for making mistakes, both your esteem and worth become eroded and damaged. Recognizing and changing distorted thinking will allow you to become less self-critical and to develop a healthier, more balanced, and compassionate view of yourself.

"Diets foster black and white thinking."

1. Black and White Thinking: As the name implies, this distortion makes you see things one of two ways—black or white. You divide your experiences, thoughts, feelings, behaviors, and decisions into one of two categories: good/bad, right/wrong, all/none, perfection/failure. Your drive for perfection demands that behaviors and appearances be perfect, or they're nothing. When you try to live within this narrow equation, it's easy to fall into the nothing zone where gray areas don't exist.

Diets foster black and white thinking. They do this by promoting the concepts of good/bad and all/none: *good* foods vs. *bad* foods; losing weight as *good* vs. stabilizing or gaining weight as *bad*; losing *all* the weight you think you need to lose or if you don't, *none* of the effort matters; and staying on a diet as *good* vs. falling off a diet as *bad*. Your whole world begins to revolve around placing what you and everyone else says and does into one of these two categories. It becomes an unconscious way of perceiving and making sense of the world. Your self-statements reflect this thinking and are usually in an "either/or" format. "Either I eat exactly what the diet says, or I've blown it." "Either I get an 'A' on this test, or I'm a bad student." "Either I get this promotion, or I'm a failure." "Either I lose weight, or no one will want to date me."

2. Generalizing: When you use a one-time incident or event to create general rules to live by, you're generalizing. Then you automatically follow those rules without testing them in different situations. They become absolute laws that dictate how you feel and think about yourself and others. Eventually, you force the information you take in to fit the rules versus seeing if the rules fit the incoming information. You hinder your growth and inclination to change with these untested rules because you follow them blindly, without exception. The way to recognize this distortion in your thinking is to look at the kinds of words you use. Do you think in terms of "always," "never," "everyone," "no one," "all," and "none?" Examples of generalizing statements might be: "I will never be thin." "Everyone thinks I'm fat." "I always make a fool of myself." "Every time I talk with my boss, I sound stupid."

3. Being in Control: When people look at how much control they have in their lives, they usually make one of two assumptions. Overcontrollers assume they have control over everything in their lives, leaving them feeling responsible for everyone's conduct in all situations. Consequently, they feel like failures for not making things happen exactly the way they imagined. No one can control another person's actions, but that doesn't stop some people from believing they can.

At the opposite extreme are the undercontrollers who assume they have *no* control over anything in their lives, leaving them feeling powerless. They believe all the power is in the hands of others, or that their lives are controlled by other forces (such as food). These individuals assign a great deal of power to food. They might make comments like: "Once I begin to eat, I can't stop myself." "The food just draws me to it."

Neither approach (overcontrol or undercontrol) takes into account that some things really are under our control and others are not. Both extremes can frustrate a person and erode self-esteem. Of the two, however, a sense of undercontrol is the most harmful because it breeds feelings of helplessness, hopelessness, and depression.

4. Global Labeling: The process of automatically stereotyping and categorizing the characteristics of yourself and others is known as global labeling, and it greatly limits your awareness of the variety of traits people possess. Most of these global labels are negative clichés that focus on appearance, thoughts, feelings, behaviors, actions, decisions, and relationships. Stereotypes reinforce negative beliefs, critical thoughts, and unempathic responses. Global labelers make statements like: "I'm a failure." "I'm a slob." "I'm dumb." "People who are fat are disgusting." "Thin people have it all."

5. Filtering: If you pay attention to only negative messages about yourself and screen out and discount other input, you're filtering. You filter by placing incoming information into one of two categories: acceptance or rejection. You accept and magnify negative messages and reject positive information. Filtering strengthens negative beliefs because the critical part of you uses this information as ammunition to confirm characteristics you've decided are bad. An example of filtering might be: When you receive your work performance review, you focus on the scores that were lower or stayed the same, while ignoring the areas in which you received a high score and praise for work well done. When you focus only on low performance scores, you reinforce the belief that you're stupid and incompetent.

6. Personalizing: Do you believe everything people say is intentionally directed toward you, as if you are the center of the universe? If you do, then you're personalizing. Other people may make comments not related to you, yet you believe they must be talking about you. You feel hurt and disappointed by what you perceive as attacks on your character. Your automatic reaction is often inappropriately defensive. For instance, your boyfriend comments on how unreliable people can be. You assume he's talking about you, so you fight with him or withdraw and become sullen. Both reactions alienate and push the other person away. Then your critic jumps in with comments about how you continually ruin relationships, and you punish yourself for screwing up once again by turning to food.

7. Self-Blame: This is blaming yourself for everything that goes wrong, even when it's not your fault. You trot out your list of personal shortcomings and go over it whenever you think you've screwed up. You then use these shortcomings to make sure you understand exactly how you messed up and take responsibility for all kinds of problems. Self-blame makes it increasingly difficult to accept yourself and have self-compassion or understanding. It also makes it easier for you to be hostile about personal flaws. Your critic constantly reminds you of how many times you make mistakes, what they are, and why it's all your fault. In defense, you reject your flaws, giving yourself an out from the continual pain of seeing all the mistakes you make. Self-blame keeps your self-esteem low by preventing good qualities from entering into your awareness. You see nothing right, only what's wrong.

8. Mind Reading: Another form of distorted thinking is believing that you can read people's mind—anticipating their thoughts, feelings, and actions. No one can read minds. What's actually happening is you're projecting your own thoughts, feelings, and beliefs onto other people. You then respond to these people as if they're thinking the same thing you are. Mostly, you project the negative aspects you perceive about yourself, and then respond to people as if they believe the same things you do about yourself. Because you think you're right, you rarely validate your interpretations. But you can damage your relationships with these leaps to unfounded conclusions.

"Catastrophizing confirms negative beliefs you
have about not deserving good things to happen."

---

9. Catastrophizing: If you constantly expect something disastrous to happen, you're catastrophizing. Just when things are going smoothly, you anticipate a catastrophe that will take away something you value or will prevent a desired outcome. Catastrophizing can actually be comforting. When disaster does strike, you feel a sense of control because you predicted it. If the outcome is less extreme than you expected, you feel happy because the full disaster did not occur. If nothing happens, you feel like you've been saved. Catastrophizing confirms negative beliefs you have about not deserving to have good things to happen. Or, it can confirm feelings you have about being bad and needing to be punished. It's easy to recognize the process. Your self-statements often sound like: "What if something bad happens just when things seem to be going so well?"

10. Shoulds: The "shoulds" come from those unbending rules you create about how you and other people need to act. These rules are idealistic and perfectionist, and when you violate them, you feel guilty, believing you're a bad person. When family members, friends, or co-workers break the rules, you become angry and disappointed with them. You attempt to change your own and other people's behaviors to match your "shoulds" list. And you make all your choices and decisions based on what you "should" be doing. Yet no one can live up to these rigid rules all the time. Even when you see this proven over and over again, you still attempt to enforce the rules. This is a method of passing on shame. Others are shamed for not living up to the rules, just as you were shamed and continue to shame yourself for not following what you think you should do.

11. Being Right: Your thinking is distorted when it becomes highly important to be right all the time. You find being wrong unthinkable, and will go to any length to prove the accuracy of your personal opinions. You base your self-esteem on being right, so it's imperative to always be perceived as having the right answers. When someone declares or proves you wrong, you feel defeated and deflated. Your relationships suffer for a number of reasons because of this need to be right. First, you don't listen to the other person. You're too busy forming a counterargument before the other person has even finished making his or her point. Because you need to be right, the other person is wrong if he or she doesn't agree with you. Second, other people wind up feeling they're wrong whenever they disagree with your opinion, and no one wants to feel wrong all the time. Their self-esteem begins to suffer and the relationship starts to erode. This is another way of passing on shame. If you were shamed about offering "wrong" opinions when growing up, most likely you unconsciously do the same thing to other people.

Shawna used all kinds of distortions to make sense of her world. She regularly perceived the world through black and white lenses—rarely did she see the middle ground. She also had a "shoulds" list a mile long that she, her husband, and two daughters had to follow. She blamed herself for everything that went wrong and needed to be in control at all times. She was exhausted by all the mind games she played. Hers was a rather unpleasant world.

Shawna's bingeing and purging were directly fueled by her mind games. Black and white thinking demanded she eat well all the time. One slip-up was cause for an all-out binge. Purging prevented any weight gain caused by the binge, or so she believed. She also made a mental list of strict rules to control her eating: no fat because she'd get heavy, no chocolate because her skin would break out, no food after six p.m., one glass of water an hour, and only one rope of licorice a day to satisfy her sweet tooth. Shawna broke every rule and then beat herself up for it. She felt incredibly stuck in her repetitive behaviors and thinking style, as if she were in a three-foot-square box with nowhere to go.

Shawna contacted me when she saw her ten-year-old daughter, Rachel, mimicking her mom's behavior with food. She felt incredibly distressed by watching Rachel skip meals, say no to candy one minute and hoard it the next, and talk about her weight all the time. We discussed how Rachel was modeling her mother's behavior. We agreed that if Shawna changed her habits, so would Rachel.

Shawna focused on two main areas: her bingeing and purging, and the unique way in which she perceived her world. The first step was to help her make changes in her eating habits. However, this would be unsuccessful without first changing her restrictive rules, black and white thinking, and need to be in control at all times. As she faced eating in a more balanced way, she saw the distortions rear their head. She learned how her distorted thinking got in the way of eating healthfully and influenced how she dealt with her children about their food habits. Shawna then began refuting the barrage of predictable judgments made by her critic. Every time she caught herself thinking critical self-statements, she forcefully challenged them, infusing factual statements.

Whenever she made a commitment to something, she gave it her all. This undertaking was no different. Over time, she whittled away the critical internal dialogue and replaced it with a more balanced way of thinking. As Shawna made changes in her eating and thinking habits, she discussed these issues with her daughter in a nonpushy way. They talked about their beliefs and food patterns. When Shawna's behaviors became more moderate, Rachel's eating habits also changed for the better.

EXAMPLES: Use these examples of distortions as a guide for when you make your list of personal distortions on the next page.

1. **Black and White Thinking:** "Either I lose 35 pounds by my 20-year high school reunion, or I'll die of embarrassment." "Either I get an 'A', or I'm a total failure."

2. **Generalizing:** "I always say stupid things when I first meet a guy." "Everyone stares at my fat legs." "I never know when to back off with my employees."

3. **Being in Control:** *Overcontrol*—"Honey, pick up the kids from soccer, stop by the store and get some french bread, and don't forget to drop by our tax man to sign the tax forms." *Undercontrol*—"I can't stop myself once I start eating chocolate."

4. **Global Labeling:** "I'm an idiot when it comes to chemistry." "Fat is disgusting."

5. **Filtering:** "I hate when I miss questions on a test. I can't seem to feel good about my performance unless I get every answer correct."

6. **Personalizing:** "I just know my boss is referring to me when she comments on how people in this office don't get her the information she requested on time."

7. **Self-Blame:** "I'm responsible for not getting the carpool to school on time. I need to get our neighbors to stop making us wait 15 minutes every day for their kids."

8. **Mind Reading:** "I just know my wife is becoming disgusted with the tire roll around my waist. I can tell because of the way she looks at me."

9. **Catastrophizing:** "I bought my first house. What if I lose my job and can't make the payments?"

10. **Shoulds:** "I should look like I did ten years ago. I hate that I don't."

11. **Being Right:** "Honey, you know I'm right. You don't want to admit it, do you?"

Assignment: Explore the ways in which you engage in distorted thinking and how your critic uses distortions to reinforce negative beliefs and to influence your behaviors.

1. Fill out *List Your Personal Distortions* to understand how your self-statements reflect the distortions and how they get played out in life.

2. Use *Refuting the Critic* to rebut the negative internal dialogue. You'll learn how to change distorted thinking by working directly with your critic. This will weaken the negative beliefs and create room for neutral and positive beliefs.

LIST YOUR PERSONAL DISTORTIONS

List the self-statement, the distortion the statement reflects, and how it gets played out in your life. For example, show how you'd play out the statement, "Honey, you know I'm right. You just don't want to admit it, do you?" Write out the complete picture, ranging from how long you're willing to fight your point, to how this affects the relationship, to how you feel about yourself, to how your partner feels.

SELF-STATEMENT	DISTORTION	HOW IT'S PLAYED OUT
1.		
2.		
3.		
4.		
5.		
6.		
7.		
8.		

CHANGING DISTORTED THINKING

The first step to changing your thinking is to consciously listen to the internal dialogue that reflects the distortions. Become aware of those critical self-statements, and then develop rebuttals to counteract the barrage of harsh internal messages. To make your rebuttals effective, it's important to incorporate the following characteristics into your self-talk. [3]

1. **Nonjudgmental:** Use factual words and phrases. Throw out any negative labels; they erode self-esteem. Judgments stop the process of empathy and compassion for yourself and others. They also separate you from yourself and from other people, making you feel either superior or inferior, depending upon the judgment.

2. **Specific:** Use terms that address specific thoughts, feelings, or behaviors instead of generalized phrases or labels.

3. **Balanced:** Include positive, neutral, and negative, yet realistic, points of view.

4. **Forceful:** Be vigilant and strong in making the rebuttal statements.

5. **Repetitive:** Say the rebuttal statement over and over again immediately after uttering a critical self-statement.

Most people who have food issues direct their distorted thinking at three areas: perceptions about the body, success vs. failure, and relationships. Below are examples of critical self-statements and rebuttals that you can make to counter the distortions.

Body-Image: The most common issue surrounding body image is weight. When you think, "I am fat," a form of *global labeling*, stop and interject a rebuttal based on the five criteria above. "My weight is _____, which is a nonjudgmental fact." Remember, you can change your beliefs and accept facts. This rebuttal is specific, balanced, and nonjudgmental. Be sure to avoid adding another critical statement to the first one, or the cycle will start all over again.

Success: The concept of success is often tied to the desire to be perfect. You equate success with never making mistakes, always knowing how to do things right, and getting everything you want. So, whenever you make an error, you beat yourself up with self-statements that reflect *black and white thinking*. "I'll never succeed," or "I'll always be a failure." To get past this, create a rebuttal that's factual and accurate but without

---

[3] McKay, M., and Fanning, P. *Self-Esteem: A Proven Program of Cognitive Techniques for Assessing, Improving, and Maintaining Self-Esteem.* Oakland, CA: New Harbinger Publications, 1987.

judgment. Let's say you left out two pages of a document you gave to your boss. The rebuttal to the critical thought might sound like this: "I know I left those two pages out of the document. I'm correcting the error by putting them in right now. Everyone forgets something at one time or another." By accepting that you made an error, you accept that you're human. This statement also fits the rebuttal criteria above.

"Making changes in your thinking requires getting to know your critical voice, which reinforces distortions in thinking."

Relationships: We all have certain ideas of how we want relationships to be. These notions shape how we respond to other people. But when we expect people to act a certain way, we're setting ourselves up for frustration and disappointment. People are what they are, and they rarely change unless they're initiating the changes. When statements reflecting the *shoulds* arise, such as, "My husband should be more diligent in his cleaning up after himself," a rebuttal can help you accept the person without judgment. The rebuttal might be: "This is how my husband cleans up. He's no different than the day I met him, and I accepted it back then. Therefore, I can accept his style and let it go." How you see your husband's behavior may also be a clue to how you believe you should be doing things.

Making changes in your thinking requires getting to know your critical voice, which reinforces distortions in thinking. Be vigilant in catching negative self-statements on an ongoing basis, then create realistic, nonhurtful, and accepting statements to replace the critical ones. This means making a daily commitment to address the ingrained messages you repeat over and over in your head.

At times, you'll feel like the critical part is winning. The critic really wants you to continue believing the old, ingrained beliefs. As you introduce healthier, more balanced, more compassionate, or neutral self-statements, and accept your perceived flaws as part of your humanness, the critic will get louder in reiterating the old beliefs. The critic is invested in having you continue using the distortions because they reinforce the negative belief system that important people in your childhood and adolescence instilled in you. That's the critic's job. To give up these negative beliefs would mean forming a new belief system—which is what will happen as you introduce new self-statements and accept your flaws.

Automatic self-statements can be changed over time when they are addressed on a continual basis. Don't be discouraged by the critic's persistence. Remember, these are beliefs, not facts. Beliefs can be changed and facts can be accepted.

REFUTING THE CRITIC

List the self-statement, the distorted thinking reflected by the statement, and the rebuttal you used to counter the critic who has been reinforcing the distortion.

SELF-STATEMENT	DISTORTION	REBUTTAL
1.		
2.		
3.		
4.		
5.		
6.		
7.		
8.		
9.		
10.		
11.		

Game 2
Perfectionism:
End the Rejection Game

Constantly striving for perfection reflects a core problem for those who struggle with unhealthy eating behaviors. The preoccupation with weight, shape, and appearance stems from the belief that physical flaws are unacceptable and must be fixed. This sense of being defective is deeply rooted in long-term feelings of inadequacy. Those feelings grow

---

"To reflect positively on parents, the child and adolescent were expected to 'look good' in many areas."

---

out of messages received during childhood and adolescence about measuring up to parental standards. To reflect positively on parents, the child and adolescent were expected to "look good" in many areas. Parents demand that their child not feel or express painful emotions, not say or do the wrong thing, always make the right choices, excel in school and extracurricular activities, never fail, and always look attractive.

One way parents demand perfection is to insist that their child have emotional control at all times. Expressing anger, fear, sadness, frustration, hurt, or disappointment is forbidden. To avoid disapproval from one or both parents, the child or adolescent decides not to show unpleasant or painful emotions. Initially, he or she may have bitten the bottom lip or pinched skin on the arm to prevent any feelings from leaking out. Depression and anxiety are likely to develop as the expression of feelings becomes effectively blocked. At some point, however, these young people discovered food had anesthetizing qualities. Bingeing, grazing, or starving became the way to cope with a wide variety of emotional experiences. Food, or the withholding of food, temporarily became a distraction from the original feelings. This denial of feelings then led to minimizing or ignoring the importance of the emotional self.

Constantly rejecting the emotional self creates an empty feeling inside a person. It becomes difficult to maintain a positive self-view because everything must be done perfectly or it's worth nothing. Since there is no perfection, and humans make mistakes all the time, these people have vast empty spaces inside that feel like nothingness.

Food fills up that hole temporarily and numbs the senses. All the feelings wind up staying in the body instead of being processed and released. If you scratched the surface of people like this, you might see years of emotions like anger, sadness, or fear that have rarely if ever been explored and released. These people condemn their emotional selves, since perfect people don't have painful feelings or bad experiences. Rejecting your emotional self is a form of self-betrayal because you want to rid yourself of the very things that make you feel alive—your emotions. Thoughts cannot create this sense of being alive like feelings can.

The message you received while growing up was that a good performance earns praise, and a better performance earns more praise. So more is better. You hope that admiration from others will sustain self-esteem and self-worth forever, but it doesn't, because you feel a constant underlying twinge of being flawed and imperfect. You work harder to attain perfection for fear someone will discover your flaws and see you for the fake that you believe yourself to be. So you strive harder for success. But your achievements don't create a lasting sense of self-worth because the good feelings dissipate until the next experience comes along to confirm that you are good. That quest for a consistent source of self-esteem from an external source (e.g., appearance, school, career, relationships) maintains the cycle of striving for perfection and success.

Negative beliefs confirm the ways in which you believe that you're flawed. The critical voice reinforces these negative beliefs every time you make a mistake, strengthening their impact. Your goal becomes doing more or doing it better—more sit-ups, longer workouts, less food, longer work hours, more classes, less sleep.

Cues From Society

The messages we all get from society also have a powerful impact. How can women value themselves when society has a hard time valuing them? Being feminine is defined in very narrow terms. Women are expected to attain physical and emotional perfection (an image prescribed by the media and the fashion industry). Yet we each inherit certain body characteristics, many of which don't mirror the look of highly paid fashion models, actresses, or dancers. Women receive all kinds of societal cues about how they should improve or alter their body shape, appearance, or moods in order to be more pleasing. This emphasis on appearance harms women and undermines their sense of self-worth because body image is an essential feature in defining identity. Body image is a complex combination of beliefs, attitudes, values, thoughts, and feelings. When women develop body hate, their self-confidence and self-esteem are eroded.

In our society, being attractive is considered so crucial for women that the media constantly bombards women with unrealistic images of how they should look. If you pay close attention to movies, television, magazines, billboards, and radio ads, you will see a pattern that encourages women to change into something more acceptable.

Media images influence both sexes and convince them that it's not only normal but also important that women purchase products to reshape their appearance. After all, the message promises that anyone can attain this beauty standard if they try hard enough or buy the right products. And when they do achieve the right look, then they will be happy, successful, and loved. Interestingly, men may be responding to similar kinds of pressures, since they're now being targeted by media campaigns that promote toned, muscular bodies.

The latest research supports a direct link between the symptoms of eating disorders and the image of women as portrayed by the media. Women who are shown media images of the thin-ideal stereotype feel stress, depression, guilt, shame, insecurity, and dissatisfaction with their own bodies. Exposure to thin models actually leads women to feel bad about their bodies and themselves, and foster the belief that women must be svelte to be attractive. Subscription to the thin-ideal increases the chance that women will engage in eating-disordered behavior. Research also shows a close relationship between dieting and eating disorders. Eating disorders are on the rise, and the single most likely culprit is people going on diets.

Objectively, you may have a fine and healthy body, yet you look in the mirror anxiously scrutinizing thighs, stomach, arms, breasts, face, and hair. Then you decide that your body isn't good enough, thin enough, or toned enough. One reason women turn to harmful eating behaviors is to control their body and to try to force it into an idealized form. Often, they take extreme steps to eliminate what they perceive as physical flaws. Dieting, starving, purging, over-exercising, and using diet pills, prescription medications, or illegal drugs become the means to attain that image. Being who you are isn't good enough. You strive to perfect the outer shell in hopes that internal suffering and self-hatred will finally stop. Yet it doesn't work. If it did, you'd be feeling great by now with all the steps you've taken to change your exterior and to whip your body into shape. Much body hate is based on a distorted perception of what the body should look like.

What you're doing isn't working. Trying to change your body by extreme measures and ignoring your emotional life by striving to feel nothing unpleasant are creating havoc. You'll enhance your self-esteem and self-worth when you change your opinion about your body versus continually trying to change your body size, shape, and weight by using harmful means that don't work. By developing a realistic view of your body and learning to accept it the way it is, you can become comfortable in your skin. The less obsessed you are with your appearance, the more satisfied you'll feel. This means giving up your perfectionist demands, critical judgments, and self-loathing, and replacing them with a sense of compassion, understanding, and acceptance of how you look.

Emotional and Mental Perfection

You'll also need to address your wish for emotional and mental perfection. Working on self-acceptance and compassion takes a daily commitment to being consciously aware of what you're feeling and thinking about yourself. This means accepting that you have a diversity of thoughts and a range of emotions. Accepting all thoughts, feelings, and bodily sensations makes them less threatening and opens the door to self-compassion. Defending against your feelings takes much more energy and stirs up more fear and anxiety than actually going through the process of experiencing them. The fear of feeling unpleasant emotions is more painful and uses much more energy than experiencing the original emotions.

"Perfection is a myth."

When your goal is perfection, you believe that perfect people don't have painful experiences, unpleasant thoughts, or unidentifiable bodily sensations. But remember, perfection is a myth. So accept your emotional and mental selves just the way they are, and you'll be honoring and respecting yourself.

Emotions act as a warning bell, telling you to attend to something in your environment or internal life that's getting stirred up. Listen to these warnings; they're instructive and will tell you what you need to pay attention to and might help you to make some changes so your life will work better.

If you catch yourself making judgments, simply note this and accept it. Then move back to the original feelings and thoughts, and work toward processing them. Many women and men have learned to accept themselves just the way they are. You can, too. It's such a relief to finally give up a judgmental attitude and to accept who you are.

To stop the cycle of perfectionism, you must take a number of steps.

1. Begin to identify and to understand the situations in which you strive for perfection. Something in these situations pushes your button and persuades you to put on your air of perfectionism. This reaction is often unconscious and automatic. Once you're aware of perfectionist attitudes and beliefs, you can monitor and refuse to act on them.

2. Stop the process of comparing yourself to other people. Every time you do this, you'll see one of two expected outcomes: either you'll be better than someone else or you'll

be worse. When you feel superior, your self-esteem is artificially pumped up. But as this feeling fades, you need to find a new situation where you can again compare yourself to someone else and win. Feeling superior doesn't last because it's not based on a continuous positive sense-of-self. Feeling inferior to someone else leads to self-denigration, which deflates self-esteem. Becoming aware of when and with whom you engage in the comparison process can help you choose to not play the game.

3. Make a list of all your qualities—strengths and flaws. Everyone has this duality. It's part of being human. Yet, you probably tend to notice only the flaws, and then reject yourself for having them. You either ignore your strengths or take them for granted. When you strive for perfection, you disown the flaws. They then haunt you because you can't get rid of them. The critic is convinced and tries to sway you into believing that only your strengths are acceptable characteristics. It uses your flaws as ammunition in the battle to lower your self-esteem. The path out of perfectionism is to accept *all* of yourself. Then the critic will have no ammunition to berate you with. Once you accept all of your qualities, the pain of being imperfect decreases. You develop a more balanced view of yourself. Plus, you will find it easier to accept other people's quirks.

4. Start today to accept yourself the way you are. You really only have two choices—either you continue to feel self-hatred for any perceived flaws, or you become self-accepting. Being *you* with all your various qualities isn't always easy, but it's more doable than attempting to be perfect. Self-acceptance doesn't mean giving up goals and dreams. You keep moving forward in life while accepting yourself just the way you are.

> *Betsy lived in the midst of perfectionism. She prided herself on showing people that she had everything under control at all times. People commented on the way she always seemed to have things go her way. Betsy made sure she looked the part. She didn't leave home without impeccably applying her makeup, fastidiously styling her hair, and dressing to the hilt. She spent hours on her appearance and checked on it throughout the day. Betsy also remained in emotional control in front of others. She refused to tell anyone anything negative about herself—creating the veneer of a perfect life. She stirred envy in others, which momentarily boosted her self-esteem. Inside, she felt like she was wilting. Mistakes she made drained every ounce of esteem from her. Striving for superiority yet feeling inferior was wreaking havoc on her sense of esteem and worth. She was burned out.*
>
> *Secretly, Betsy binged and purged to cope with the stresses related to work and relationships. Underneath all that makeup and fashionable attire was a person who was fatigued from food abuse and racked with*

painful emotions that had been suppressed for years. Betsy felt anxious much of the time and used food to turn off the spigot of anxiety.

Betsy consulted me when her life felt beyond her control. She was having a harder time presenting herself as a perfect being, plus the eating behaviors and unresolved emotions were taking their toll. We devised a plan in which Betsy made changes that included altering eating habits, reducing the purging behavior, introducing exercise as a method of stress reduction, and identifying, understanding, and processing her feelings.

The next step was to address Betsy's need for perfectionism. In exploring why she must be seen as perfect and in control at all times, she described a life in which she earned a great deal of praise from her whole family when she appeared perfect. She learned how to present herself in such a way as to elicit praise and envy from others. She valued the superficial, rarely searching for the depth and meaning in life.

Betsy began her search by looking at aspects of the self she disowned—her flaws and unpleasant emotions. She then consciously worked on two areas: not comparing herself to media images or people she perceived as superior to her, and accepting those parts of herself she had previously discarded. Initially, she found this quite uncomfortable. Once she became more accepting of those characteristics, she began to feel more of her feelings and to express them to others. She started with her boyfriend and best friend, eventually moving on to her family.

Betsy's anxiety level alternately increased and decreased depending on what she was working on. She felt quite anxious when she expressed her feelings to others, letting them see behind the wall of perfection. With practice and time, the anxiety eventually subsided. When she experienced her emotions, she felt less anxious because she wasn't converting unwanted feelings into anxiety, as she had in the past. Betsy emerged from the fog of perfectionism, living a more balanced and full life, and truly liking herself more than she ever thought possible.

Assignment: Focus on why you consistently strive for perfection and how you keep yourself from feeling good about yourself. You'll learn how to stop the cycle of perfection and make peace with imperfection.

1. Use *List How You Strive for Perfection* to see where, when, and how perfectionism permeates your behaviors and actions.

2. Fill out *The Comparison Process* to see with whom you compare yourself, whether you felt superior or inferior, and how you stopped comparing yourself to them.

3. List your *Strengths and Flaws* to begin accepting all of your characteristics.

4. Create a list of *Accepting Self-Statements* to counteract the critical statements you make about your perceived flaws.

LIST HOW YOU STRIVE FOR PERFECTION

List where, when, and how perfectionism permeates your behaviors and actions.

WHERE AND WHEN	HOW YOU STRIVE FOR PERFECTION
1.	
2.	
3.	
4.	
5.	
6.	
7.	
8.	
9.	
10.	
11.	
12.	
13.	
14.	
15.	
16.	
17.	
18.	

THE COMPARISON PROCESS

Make a list of all the people to whom you compared yourself throughout the week. List the feelings this created—superiority or inferiority. Then note whether or not you were able to stop the comparison process by recognizing what you were doing and making a conscious decision to stop.

PERSON	FEELINGS	HOW YOU STOPPED THE COMPARISON PROCESS
1.		
2.		
3.		
4.		
5.		
6.		
7.		
8.		
9.		
10.		
11.		
12.		
13.		

STRENGTHS AND FLAWS

The self has two main sides—characteristics you consider desirable and those you don't. You stop the cycle of striving for perfection when you accept your full self, both the strengths and the flaws. List your strengths and flaws.

STRENGTHS

1. _____
2. _____
3. _____
4. _____
5. _____
6. _____
7. _____
8. _____
9. _____
10. _____
11. _____
12. _____
13. _____
14. _____
15. _____
16. _____
17. _____
18. _____

FLAWS

1. _____
2. _____
3. _____
4. _____
5. _____
6. _____
7. _____
8. _____
9. _____
10. _____
11. _____
12. _____
13. _____
14. _____
15. _____
16. _____
17. _____
18. _____

ACCEPTING SELF-STATEMENTS

Create a list of accepting self-statements to counteract the critical self-statements about your perceived flaws. Create nonjudgmental, specific, balanced, forceful, and repetitive statements (refer to the five steps to correct distorted thinking, p. 145).

ACCEPTING SELF-STATEMENTS

1. _____

2. _____

3. _____

4. _____

5. _____

6. _____

7. _____

8. _____

9. _____

10. _____

11. _____

12. _____

13. _____

14. _____

15. _____

16. _____

17. _____

18. _____

Game 3
Watchful Eye:
Take Off the "Mask" and Be Yourself

Everyone pays attention to how they act, to some degree. Some people monitor and adjust their behaviors according to the situation, whereas others don't. People who have a "watchful eye" are highly concerned about social appropriateness, paying particular attention to the facial expressions and presentation of others. They take these signals as cues to guide their behavior. Because every situation is different, those with a watchful eye alter their behaviors to fit the circumstances. They strive to make sure other people see them in the way they want to be perceived—nice, pleasant, thoughtful, kind, generous, even-tempered, patient, loving, or tolerant.

"You avoid criticism from others and from your internal critic by making sure your behavior pleases others."

The behaviors and actions of people with a watchful eye have a chameleon-like quality, varying from situation to situation. Having a watchful eye makes being true to the self difficult. It also makes it hard to consistently know the self because actions change depending on the situation. How confusing!

Negative beliefs and critical internal dialogue promote the development of a watchful eye. You learned early on that it pleased your parents and other significant persons when you did or said the right thing because they praised you. When you didn't adapt to the situation and made mistakes, you were criticized and judged. Now, you try to figure out what other people expect of you so there's less chance of doing or saying something inappropriate and, therefore, fewer conflicts. You avoid criticism from others and from your internal critic by making sure your behavior pleases others. It feels much safer to wear a "mask" to hide your true self than to be authentic and vulnerable. The mask makes it necessary to adopt diverse behaviors to fit in, no matter what the situation. The mask changes depending on where the wearer is and what is happening. It serves as a protective device against people who don't like the real you and, therefore, prompts people-pleasing behaviors. When the mask slips because you didn't successfully monitor your behaviors, you fear someone will see something horrible about you—your flaws.

"Deep and honest relationships don't develop when thoughts, feelings, and behaviors are modified to please other people and avoid conflict."

Some people monitor their thoughts, feelings, and behaviors only with people they see as significant; others do it with everyone. Most people wear their mask when they deal with feelings about other people. It seems too risky to take a stand on an issue or to express certain kinds of emotions considered negative—anger, sadness, frustration, fear, disappointment, or hurt. It becomes much easier to avoid situations that may lead to confrontation. The watchful eye makes sure you adjust your behaviors to be pleasing. Yet deep and honest relationships don't develop when thoughts, feelings, and behaviors are modified to please other people and avoid conflict.

We've all met them—people who are guided by their own opinions about themselves, not really caring what others think. Individuals without a mask dress, act, think, and talk similarly across situations. There may be slight variations, however, they don't watch their behaviors and reactions, nor change them to please others. There is a commitment to attitudes and values, using them to guide their behaviors.

By taking off the mask and not engaging the watchful eye, you have an opportunity to get to know yourself. You become more self-trusting and authentic when you're in touch with and express the whole you—all aspects of yourself. Your true self is reflected in your strengths and flaws. You are a composite of these characteristics. When you own all your traits, you have an idea of what your true self looks like.

You need to take two steps to decrease your use of the watchful eye and to stop wearing your mask:

1. Assess where, when, and with whom you alter your behaviors to fit the situation. Pay attention to who you're doing this for and in which situations it happens. Once you can clearly see what you're doing, then you can make the necessary changes.

2. Take the risk of being authentic and true to yourself. This includes being honest with yourself and others about what you feel and think, what you believe, and the attitudes you hold. It also means not changing your behaviors to fit into situations because you believe the situation warrants it, but acting in a way that is true to the self. Your behaviors will be less wishy-washy, and you'll have a greater sense of who you are.

> *"People who are accustomed to your people-pleasing style*
> *may be caught off guard when you begin to be yourself."*

This doesn't necessarily mean sharing everything with everyone all the time. Discretion as to what you say and when you say it can be valuable. Being honest, truthful, and trusting of yourself is highly important; then you can be that way with others you deem safe. Place your trust only in people who prove themselves to be trustworthy. Don't offer information that will come back to haunt or harm you in some way. Do share when it will further communication and connections with others.

People who are accustomed to your people-pleasing style may be caught off guard when you begin to be yourself. They may be uncomfortable because you were so easy to get along with when you adapted to their expectations. Explain to them what you're doing and why. Your true friends and loyal supporters will accept the changes you're making and will see the rewards—a deepening in their relationship with you. You'll also know when to give and to do it freely of your own accord, not because you think you should or because it's expected of you.

The critic is bound to be harsh and judgmental when you take off the mask and don't monitor your behaviors. The critic has used this to protect you from confrontations with others and any unpleasant feelings that may result. The critic has also kept you from knowing your true self. Be vigilant in not giving in to the critic. The healthy voice will prevail.

Part of what you'll be doing is trial and error in learning how to be in touch with your true self and how to be authentic in your interactions with others. When you begin the process of getting in touch with your true self, try it in situations that are not very threatening—meaning ones where there are few consequences to being yourself. Once you've mastered the easier situations, move on to more difficult ones. Experiences with family members are often more stressful and threatening than others. If this is true for you, you may want to experiment and practice with other people and situations before you do this with your family.

> *Susan was hyperaware of her environment. In an instant, she could read what was happening in a room full of people and decide the best way to act. She was good! Susan learned this skill from monitoring family members' changing moods and altering her behavior to fit the situation. She feared any type of conflict and prided herself on her ability to skirt confrontation.*
>
> *Susan also felt confused and empty much of the time because she spent so much energy focusing on what other people wanted from and expected of her. She lost the connection with herself and grew tired of*

feeling lost and frustrated that people didn't try to please her as much as she tried to please them.

Susan originally came to see me for her issues with food. She ate all the time. She did free-lance work at home and found herself either in the kitchen munching on food, or taking a bowlful of popcorn or candy to her desk, where she could scoop out one handful after another. Susan was able to retrain herself to eat meals and snacks with time in between. Plus, she modified her food choices to lower-fat, higher-fiber foods—fruits, vegetables, and grains. In addition, she ate her favorite foods—popcorn and candy—in one-serving-size amounts as part of the meal or as a snack. She stopped keeping a bowl of food at her work table.

Susan also wanted to address the incredible sense of emptiness she felt and to stop being a chameleon where others were concerned. For years she had changed her behavior with her family and husband and at work-related and social functions. She worried about what others would think and feared that conflicts would arise if she took care of herself first. Susan's initial step was to get to know herself—what she felt, thought, believed, and why she acted the way she did. The process of defining these qualities led Susan to gain more of a sense of herself, and the emptiness began to fade. Once she was able to identify her true feelings on a regular basis, she worked to be true to them. She vowed to listen to her internal guidance system and to drop her watchful eye. She listened to the whispers of intuition that she had ignored for years.

Susan also made mistakes. She wasn't always as sensitive or diplomatic about meeting her own needs. She ruffled feathers and made social faux pas at parties. In the beginning it was quite stressful, and at times embarrassing, to act in accordance with her beliefs—until she got the hang of it. Once she reaped the rewards of inner satisfaction from being true to herself and seeing that she didn't lose her family or husband, Susan emerged a more whole person.

Assignment: Assess how you monitor your behavior and adjust it to fit the situation. Fill out *How You Use the Watchful Eye* to become familiar with where, when, and with whom you adapt your behaviors. Then discover techniques for *Decreasing the Use of the Watchful Eye* by being authentic and true to yourself.

HOW YOU USE THE WATCHFUL EYE

Become familiar with where, when, and with whom you adapt your behaviors to fit a situation. Think about how you present yourself at work and work-related activities, social functions, church, school, meetings, etc. Pay attention to how you act with family members, partners, friends, coworkers, authority figures, and acquaintances. List the situation and/or person for whom you change your behaviors and note the mask you wear (how you act) at that time.

SITUATION/PERSON	MASK (HOW YOU ACT)
1.	
2.	
3.	
4.	
5.	
6.	
7.	
8.	
9.	
10.	
11.	
12.	
13.	
14.	
15.	
16.	

DECREASING THE USE OF THE WATCHFUL EYE

You needn't abandon the use of your watchful eye completely. In some situations it may be necessary and even helpful. However, in general it's important to be you regardless of the situation or who you're with. This means taking some risks and walking through your fears about people rejecting you. When other people's opinions about you don't matter very much, changing your behaviors to please them becomes unnecessary. You become authentic with yourself and others. You'll also know when to be giving and when to give freely because you choose to, not because it is expected of you.

Try it out. Pick a situation from the previous list. The next time that situation arises, behave in a manner that reflects being true to yourself. Record the situation, behaviors that mirror your true self, and how it felt to be true to yourself. Start small, with situations and people who aren't very threatening. When the critic chimes in with judgments, refute him or her, using the techniques you've already learned.

SITUATION	TRUE SELF BEHAVIORS	HOW IT FELT
1.		
2.		
3.		
4.		
5.		
6.		
7.		

Game 4
Nonassertiveness:
Learn to Speak Your Mind

Nonassertiveness is an acquired behavior. Many people learn from their parents and others how to be passive, which means ignoring their thoughts, feelings, and rights to be accepted by others. Meeting one's own needs becomes less important than meeting someone else's. By giving in to other people's wishes and demands, you avoid conflicts, which is why being nonassertive is so seductive. When you show more concern for someone other than yourself, it's self-betrayal because you don't allow yourself the full expression of your thoughts and feelings.

"You betray yourself when you don't stick up for yourself."

In relationships, people exhibit three different styles of behaviors:

Passive: Behaving passively means doing what you're told, not expressing thoughts or feelings, avoiding taking a stand, and allowing others to push you around no matter how uncomfortable it feels. People behave passively to avoid being criticized, to prevent a conflict, or to be liked by everyone. The payoff for passive behavior is that it reduces your chances of being rejected. The downside is feeling angry or resentful when someone takes advantage of you because you know that you've allowed it. You betray yourself when you don't stick up for yourself.

Aggressive: Behaving aggressively includes screaming, attacking, blaming, fighting, threatening someone, or acting in a way that conveys little respect for the other person. People behave aggressively to feel more in control and to ward off feelings of insecurity or fear. The payoff for aggressive behavior is that no one pushes you around. The downside is that people won't want to spend time with you or will be afraid of you.

Assertive: Behaving assertively means expressing thoughts, feelings, beliefs, and opinions in a socially appropriate manner. You communicate respect for yourself and for others, while protecting your personal rights. You refuse to tolerate the passive or aggressive behaviors of others. You take actions with your own best interest in mind, while not allowing others to take advantage of you. The payoff is getting what you want without being offensive. Being passive or aggressive doesn't work for long. Being assertive does.

"If someone rejects you because you're assertive, that says a great deal about the other person, doesn't it?"

Negative beliefs and critical internal dialogue demand that you be liked by everyone. How can you be assertive when you believe other people matter more than you? When you trust that your thoughts and feelings are all right, you'll be more willing to express them and to be true to them. If someone rejects you because you're assertive, that says a great deal about the other person, doesn't it?

Every relationship involves certain acceptable rights. You have the right to express your reactions in a way that conveys respect for yourself and for other people. Listed below are some of your assertive rights.

Eleven Assertive Rights:

1. You have the right to own and accept all your beliefs, opinions, thoughts, feelings, decisions, and choices.

2. You have the right to experience and express your pain.

3. You have the right to ask for help or emotional support when you need it.

4. You have the right to make mistakes and be to accountable for them.

5. You have the right to be illogical and experiment when making decisions, without justifying your actions.

6. You have the right not to take responsibility for or worry about other people's problems.

7. You have the right to change your mind.

8. You have the right to say, "No."

9. You have the right to say, "I don't know."

10. You have the right to say, "I don't understand."

11. You have the right to say, "I don't care."

William used to describe his boss as a pain in the neck—a man who was extremely demanding and who rarely provided strokes for a job well done. William considered resigning from his job as assistant hotel manager, but he needed the money. He did grunt work, even though it wasn't part of his job description, passively accepting the assignments anyway. William finally reached the breaking point and contacted me when he was on the verge of walking off the job.

In addition, William wanted to address his eating pattern of one large meal at the end of the workday, a habit that had put too much weight on him. He saw a direct link between the stress of his job and how he ate. In the evening, he numbed out in a major way by consuming the equivalent of two meals plus dessert. He starved himself during the day in hopes of losing weight. But it wasn't working—he was getting heavier. The plan was to spread out the amount of food to three meals a day and to cut down on fast foods. He was able to follow the plan and, with practice and time, the weight eventually dropped.

William needed to focus on his work situation as well as his food and weight issues. So while he was making changes in how and what he ate, he also addressed his passive style of communication. He learned early on that asking for what he wanted got him in trouble. It's perhaps no accident that his boss reminded him of his father—demanding and unrelenting in his criticism. William criticized himself much like his father and boss did.

William addressed two interrelated areas. He learned how to counter his own critical voice and how to be more assertive. He focused on refuting his critic every time it reared its head, and on really grasping the instilled beliefs that led him to be so hypercritical and passive. He then took an active roll in making assertive statements, and meaning them. He started small—with Max, his best friend since the third grade. He practiced on Max and asked for feedback on his emerging assertive style. He then moved on to being assertive with his boss. Again he started out small, being assertive on issues that had little consequence. He moved on to assertively refusing to do grunt work, backing it up with an alternative solution—and the sparks flew. But William held his ground, staying rational, cool-headed, and direct. His boss blew steam, then calmed down, and William got his way. Was he ever surprised! Even though he didn't always act assertively, he did so more and more. His confidence began to grow, as did his job satisfaction.

Assignment: Read your *Eleven Assertive Rights*, take the *Nonassertiveness Test*, and learn how to develop *Assertive Behavior* in your communication with others. Use the *Becoming Assertive* chart to assess old behaviors, new behaviors, and how it feels to be assertive.

NONASSERTIVENESS TEST

Below are questions for assessing nonassertive behavior. Check (✓) the ones that apply.

1. Do you outwardly agree with people when you really don't agree? _____

2. Are you swayed by other people's opinions? _____

3. Are you compliant with other people's wishes or demands when it's not in your own best interest or you don't want to comply? _____

4. Do you seek praise by conforming to other people's expectations of you? _____

5. Do you find other people's opinions more important than your own? _____

6. Do you discount your thoughts, feelings, or opinions? _____

7. Do you avoid conflicts? _____

8. Do you avoid other people's anger? _____

9. Do you believe you shouldn't have the feelings you do? _____

10. Do you judge your reactions as oversensitive or stupid? _____

11. Do you believe you should have only pleasant feelings? _____

12. Do you feel guilty for disagreeing with others? _____

13. Do you believe the best way to keep relationships going is to give in? _____

14. Do you avoid speaking up even when you disagree with something someone is saying? _____

15. Do you believe men like passive, compliant women? _____

16. Do you believe women like passive, compliant men? _____

Scoring: Give yourself 1 point for each question you have checked, then compute your total score. The score indicates the severity of your problems with assertiveness.

1.	Mild	=	1 – 4
2.	Moderate	=	5 – 8
3.	Serious	=	9 – 12
4.	Severe	=	13 – 16

Note: The Nonassertiveness Test is not intended to be used as a diagnostic measurement, but as an opportunity for self-exploration and awareness. You can use this test to examine your level of assertiveness. You can gain insight from this information, and then create change.

ASSERTIVE BEHAVIOR

There are a number of steps to take when changing from being passive or aggressive to being assertive. You need to develop an awareness of what's happening in your conversations with other people. Then you can learn new behaviors. These new behaviors will direct the way you interact. By being assertive, you'll increase your communications and connections with others, which will make your relationships more mutually satisfying.

Steps to becoming assertive include:

1. Choose a place that's comfortable and safe to deal with the interaction or conflict.

2. Clearly express your thoughts, feelings, beliefs, and attitudes using "I" statements rather than "you" statements to convey that you own your reactions. For example, "I feel angry," instead of, "You made me angry."

3. Avoid disclaiming or minimizing what you say.

4. Ask the other person if they understand your point of view.

5. Communicate what you think about the conversation.

6. Tell how you feel about what's happening in the interaction.

7. Maintain eye contact, project your voice, speak clearly, and smile only when you mean it.

8. Raise your voice, repeat a phrase, tell the person you would like to continue before they respond, or raise your hand to stop them when they try to interrupt your assertive expression.

9. Ask questions or request that they clarify or elaborate their point when you feel confused about what they're saying.

10. Tell the other person that you will not continue the conversation if they become verbally abusive, and you will only continue when the behavior has stopped.

11. Say "thank you" for a compliment without justifying, minimizing, or discounting the comment.

12. Don't expect the other person to change drastically from the way they have been in the past, even though you are becoming more assertive.

BECOMING ASSERTIVE

Learning to be assertive takes lots of practice, and it's important to work at becoming comfortable with acting in an assertive manner. When the opportunity arises to practice new behaviors, take the chance. Create a list of the situations, the old passive or aggressive behaviors, the new assertive behaviors, and how it felt to be assertive. This will help you see the successes that can result from taking care of yourself.

SITUATION	OLD BEHAVIOR	NEW BEHAVIOR	FEELING
1.			
2.			
3.			
4.			
5.			
6.			
7.			

Game 5
Anticipation:
It's Time to Live in the Here and Now

Consider how often your mind drifts from present-moment experiences to future events, wishes, and dreams. Your thoughts automatically focus on how much better life will be once certain factors change—be it your weight, appearance, relationships, finances, or job opportunities. You believe that once certain circumstances improve, you'll be happy.

"When you expect life to be different instead of appreciating all that is happening now, you criticize yourself for not having attained what you think you should have."

This mindset can make life seem very empty because you ignore or discount the pleasant and realistic aspects of the present.

When you expect life to be different, instead of accepting and appreciating all that you have today, you end up harshly criticizing yourself for not having attained the things you believe you should have by now. To identify this style of thinking in yourself, listen for self-statements you make in a "When I . . . , then I . . ." form. A classic example is, "When I get thin, then I will . . . ." Anything can fit into the blank: "like myself," "find someone to love," "be happy," "get a partner," "attain financial success," "achieve career success," and so on. Notice that the desired event has *yet* to happen. And when and if it does, it rarely has the impact you believe it will. The pleasure it brings fades, and a new anticipation is set in motion.

Buying in to the diet mentality keeps you in the anticipation trap. Think about all the diets you've tried and all the weight you've lost. Have they created any long-term happiness? If they did, why didn't the weight stay off?

Continually striving to eliminate the bad or painful aspects of yourself and your life makes it difficult to accept things as they are. When you strive to be perfect, you can't allow anything in life to be negative. You set goals to change things in the future with the hope of feeling better about yourself, which makes it impossible for your life to be satisfying right now. When the anticipated change finally occurs, happiness and joy don't seem to last long.

The whole anticipation game is based on the belief that if you finally reach perfection with things easily going your way, then life will become and remain good, with no problems, no failures, no pain. You make up your mind that you cannot be happy until then. However, the pleasure of reaching the desired goal isn't strong enough to alter your ingrained negative beliefs. They will eventually rear their heads and let you know that you're still messing up, not measuring up, or not doing or being enough.

Live in the Here and Now

When you live in anticipation, you create goals to change something in the future and ignore the present. The way to break this cycle is to begin living in the here and now. After all, it's all you have. The past is gone and the future has yet to arrive. All any of us *really* have is this moment in time. When you dislike yourself now, today feels miserable. To feel satisfied, you need to accept yourself and your life the way they are.

"Living in the moment takes practice."

When you approve of yourself and your life circumstances the way they are today, while continuing to address the changes you need to make, positive feelings emerge. You've already discovered the alternative doesn't work. When there's little or no self-acceptance of the qualities you've been attempting to disown, negative feelings about the self abound. This doesn't mean you give up your goals, however, you don't predicate your happiness on changing things. You can be productive and accept yourself at the same time.

You probably play the anticipation game in many different areas of your life. Weight and appearance are usually high on the list, but there are also other areas. For example, it's easy to live in anticipation if you're in school and looking forward to finishing a semester or graduating, waiting to get engaged or married, ready to have children, changing jobs, or moving to a new city. It can even be a moment-to-moment experience of watching the clock and wanting a class, the workday, a plane ride, or bad date to end. When you wish your time away, you've surrendered whatever opportunity there was to get something meaningful out of the experience. By recognizing the areas in which you play the anticipation game, you'll start to see where you lack acceptance of yourself and of your life. You need to accept what you've been rejecting or ignoring and reinforce the positive.

Living in the moment takes practice. It's so easy to drift off and think about other things besides what you're doing right now. This habit will take time to break and may even seem impossible, but being aware of what you're doing can help bring you back to the present. Then work on accepting yourself just the way you are in that moment. Be patient. When you devote time toward both processes, it will eventually get easier. You'll begin to feel better about yourself and your life now.

Catherine felt excited about her latest diet and couldn't wait till she lost 30 pounds. She would then do all the things she'd been putting off for years. She'd hated her body for so long, scrutinizing every inch, criticizing all her flaws. This was going to be the diet that finally worked. She anticipated that when she lost the weight, she would be so happy—just like her law partner, Maggy. Maggy was thin and happy. Catherine was sure that thinness was what made Maggy's life happy. She failed to realize that Maggy was experiencing a lot of personal problems. All Catherine could see was a thin body.

She dieted for one month and lost ten pounds. But then she felt so hungry and deprived that she wound up bingeing for three days in a row. She gained back seven pounds and felt thoroughly disgusted with herself. She loathed her body even more and sunk into a pit of depression. Finally, she decided she needed to stop banking on losing weight to make her life better.

When Catherine consulted me, her first reaction was, "You're suggesting that I accept the way I look. I can't imagine liking myself at this weight or being happy where I am right now." It took her weeks to see that her joy and happiness had nothing to do with how much she weighed. She looked at pictures taken five years ago during a Club Med trip to Tahiti— when she was 25 pounds lighter. She wasn't happy then, either. As a matter of fact, she felt fat, ugly, and miserable. This convinced Catherine that her size was inconsequential in the equation of what brings her joy.

She combined accepting self-statements with a diet-free approach to weight management. She chipped away at the self-loathing she had experienced for so long. Self-acceptance came long before any changes in her appearance. As the weeks went by, she became more appreciative of all her personal attributes, and she didn't let her weight stop her from doing the things she wanted to do. Then, by eating three meals a day and allowing herself the goodies she craved, within moderation, she felt more comfortable with food. Eating well and biking through the fields behind her house eventually altered her metabolism, and she slowly lost weight. Catherine had to admit that the path to her happiness had nothing to do with being thin.

Assignment: Discover why you live in anticipation of the future and how to redirect your focus to being in the moment. List *The Anticipation Game* you play with yourself. Learn techniques for *Changing the Anticipation Game* and *Living in the Moment.*

THE ANTICIPATION GAME

List the anticipation games you play, what negative beliefs about yourself they reinforce, and what part of yourself you're rejecting. Begin to notice how little self-acceptance you have in these particular areas. For example, if you say to yourself, "When I get thin, I will find a boyfriend and be happy," you're reinforcing the belief that you're unlovable because of your weight. What you're rejecting is your body—wanting to change it so that you can be loved.

WHEN I . . . THEN I . . .	NEGATIVE BELIEF	WHAT YOU ARE REJECTING
1.		
2.		
3.		
4.		
5.		
6.		
7.		
8.		
9.		

CHANGING THE ANTICIPATION GAME

You need to own and accept the parts of yourself you're trying to disown because your belief system doesn't approve of them. If you can accept them now, you won't be living in the future, waiting for your life to get better once these things change. The way to accept yourself and your life is to use accepting self-statements. Start with the previous example of, "When I get thin, then I will find a boyfriend and be happy." Replace the statement of anticipation with accepting self-statements that have the qualities of being nonjudgmental, specific, and balanced. An example might be, "I accept that I don't have a boyfriend and accept that I want one. I also accept my body the way it is because it's not going to change into something I desire at this very moment. I accept that sometimes I feel unlovable. It's a feeling not a fact, though. I am okay today without a boyfriend." Write down the anticipation games you play and the self-accepting statements you'll replace them with.

WHEN I . . . , THEN I . . .	ACCEPTING SELF-STATEMENTS
1.	
2.	
3.	
4.	
5.	
6.	
7.	
8.	
9.	
10.	
11.	
12.	
13.	
14.	

LIVING IN THE MOMENT

Every time you catch yourself focusing on something other than what you're thinking, feeling, and doing now, you're missing the only experience you have available to you. Practice living in the moment by consciously redirecting your attention back to what is happening right now. Notice what you're experiencing now, why you're drifting away (e.g., the future is more important; you don't like what you're going through now; if you don't focus on the future, you won't succeed), and how it feels to live in the here and now.

CURRENT EXPERIENCE	REASONS FOR DRIFTING AWAY	FEELINGS ABOUT THE "NOW"
1.		
2.		
3.		
4.		
5.		
6.		
7.		
8.		
9.		

3 - 8

Affirm Yourself Daily:
What You Say Can Heal You

Your positive and negative internal dialogue has a tremendous influence on how you regard yourself. When you continually repeat critical self-statements based on negative beliefs, what choice do you have but to accept them as real? You must change both the beliefs and the self-statements.

"Affirmations allow you to accept all the flaws you've been rejecting as unacceptable."

Affirmations can be an effective way to counter your negative internal dialogue. They offer alternative ways of viewing a wide variety of personality traits often labeled as negative. Affirmations allow you to accept all the flaws you've been rejecting as unacceptable. As long as you consider personal flaws "bad," you'll disown them. You must accept the whole of you. By owning and accepting all of your characteristics, you can recognize your humanness and learn to like yourself, creating a sense of inner peace.

Thanks to your desire to be perfect, you often overlook your good qualities because you don't see them as being good enough (i.e., perfect) or you take them for granted, not noticing them. Therefore, it's important to recognize and affirm your positive characteristics. You might consider many of your thoughts, feelings, and behaviors unacceptable because you consider them flaws or weaknesses. But these, too, must be affirmed as part of yourself. This will make them more neutral in your eyes rather than horrible and disgusting. Because your attitude about yourself affects how you feel and think about yourself, the attitude needs to change. But you needn't give up goals or stop making changes. It's easier to change things that aren't working when you recognize them and accept them as part of yourself.

Create positive or neutral self-statements that you can believe about yourself. When you begin making these kinds of statements, your critic will become louder. Ingrained negative thoughts will automatically pop up to counter the new self-statements.

> *"The need to eat to fill the emptiness decreases
> as self-knowledge and acceptance increase."*

Talk with your critic. Tell him or her why you're doing this—to change negative beliefs and attitudes and accept the full you, including all your strengths and flaws. Let your critic know you are not trying to get rid of it, you're just redirecting its energies. In other words, you're accepting your humanness. Restate the affirmations over and over again. When you can accept who you are, you'll feel a great sense of relief. Those critical self-judgments will decrease and a sense of your complete self will spring up instead. This counteracts any sense of internal emptiness because you're filling yourself with information about yourself. The need to eat to fill the emptiness decreases as self-knowledge and acceptance increase.

To be effective, self-affirmations must:

- Affirm who you are now, not who you want to be in the future.

- Affirm what you want to happen now, not what you desire in the future.

- Affirm what you want, not what you don't want.

- Affirm your acceptance of your strengths and flaws.

- Affirm the results you desire if you want to make reasonable changes in your life.

In addition, you must make a commitment to:

- Say self-affirmations on a daily basis.

- Give the self-affirmations time to work without setting up an artificial timeline to change your thinking. Changing beliefs and attitudes can be slow. New ways of thinking and feeling unfold over time.

- Let the self-affirmation manifest itself in its own way. The form may be different than you expected. Accept whatever comes.

- Imagine the desired result of the self-affirmation in your head, as if it's happening right now.

- Make self-affirmations for today, with the option of changing your mind tomorrow. This kind of permission helps you to focus on one day at a time and doesn't make you feel boxed in trying something forever.

- Write down the self-affirmations on sticky notes. Place them where you can see them every day to remind yourself of what you want to affirm.

An effective way to consistently remind yourself of self-affirmations is to make a recording of the statements. They can either be recorded in your own voice or someone else's. Some people feel it's more believable to hear their own voice; others respond better to someone else's voice. Repeat each affirmation five times on the tape. Listen to the tape at least once a day for a minimum of three months, and longer if you desire.

Marie was tired of hating her body. She wanted to accept her body's size and shape. In high school, she had dreamed of growing to five feet, nine inches. She never made it past five feet, three inches. For years she had envied women who were tall and slender. Marie had a medium-size bone structure, so with her slight stature, she looked more square than reedlike. She had tried just about everything to look taller and leaner, but nothing worked for very long. She had tried all types of diets, spent years rigorously working out, and wore bone-crushing stiletto heels. Short of severe starvation and a stretching machine, she wasn't going to attain her idealized image.

She consulted me to help her come to terms with her appearance. We discussed the reality of how she looked and focused on her accepting her appearance. Within months of practicing realistic affirmations, refuting her critic, and changing her narrowly defined beliefs, Marie began noticing a change in how she saw herself. She felt much more positive about all her characteristics and came to accept her height and build. She eventually decided that she didn't have to keep whipping her body into something it would never become—and she gave up wearing three-inch heels. The relief was incredible. She actually started liking her unique looks, appreciating what she had, rather than hating herself for what she didn't have.

Assignment: *Creating Affirmations* is an effective tool to counteract negative internal dialogue. You'll learn how to create powerful *Affirmations* that reduce critical self-statements and build positive self-talk.

CREATING AFFIRMATIONS

To begin creating positive and neutral feelings about yourself, you need to experience self-acceptance. This means affirming daily that the whole of you is acceptable just the way you are. What you're telling yourself is that nothing needs to change to be okay.

"I accept myself exactly the way I am today. I may change my mind tomorrow, but for today, I accept myself."

This includes your weight, shape, and appearance. In the beginning, it's not necessary to like, love, or appreciate these disowned qualities—the aspects of yourself that you perceive as imperfect or flawed and that must be ignored or cast aside. You need only to be accepting of them. Once beliefs change and you start accepting yourself, positive feelings will follow. You're countering the critical internal dialogue that only has power as long as you believe it. Give yourself the option of changing your mind tomorrow, but, for now, commit to affirming yourself today. Do the same with your feelings. Painful or unpleasant feelings are easy to disown, deny, or avoid. By accepting them, you create the opportunity to feel them and move through the experience, which releases them. Listed below are examples of different kinds of affirmations.

Self-Acceptance Affirmation: "I accept myself exactly how I am today. I may change my mind tomorrow, but for today, I accept myself."

Self-Acceptance Affirmation for Feelings: "I accept how I'm feeling right now. It may not be particularly comfortable, it may even be painful, yet I accept how I feel at this moment. I may decide to ignore my feelings tomorrow, but for today, I am accepting them."

Self-Acceptance Affirmation for Body-Image: "I accept my body the way it is today. I may decide to change my mind tomorrow and hate my body, but for today, I accept it."

Self-Acceptance Affirmation for Making Mistakes: "I accept myself even though I made a mistake. Everyone makes mistakes from time to time. I may choose to hate myself tomorrow for any mistakes I make then, but for today, I accept that I made a mistake and I am still okay."

You can create affirmations to address all kinds of negative beliefs that lead you to reject parts of yourself. Negative beliefs and the corresponding critical self-statements can affect many areas of your life including work, school, relationships, extracurricular activities, and idle time. Create a list of affirmations that address the specific areas in which you find yourself disowning or rejecting pieces of who you are.

AFFIRMATIONS

Create a list of affirmations you can say every day. Use the list of characteristics that make an affirmation effective. By fitting the affirmation into the format on the previous page, you can accept anything.

AFFIRMATIONS

1. _____

2. _____

3. _____

4. _____

5. _____

6. _____

7. _____

8. _____

9. _____

10. _____

11. _____

12. _____

13. _____

14. _____

15. _____

16. _____

17. _____

18. _____

3 - 9

Progressive Relaxation:
The Ultimate Stress Buster

People who struggle with unhealthy eating patterns often have a difficult time relaxing. They're constantly directing their thoughts toward doing something productive. Downtime finally comes only after they collapse into bed at the end of the day. Learning to relax adds a sense of balance and enhances a person's quality of life. As valuable as it is to accomplish tasks, it's equally important to know how to take time off and relax. The psyche needs time to recuperate from the stresses and strains of everyday life.

"When you learn to relax, you have time to tune in to your body and listen to what it has to say."

Progressive Relaxation[4] is a proven technique that helps counteract tension. Relaxation and physiological tension are incompatible, so when you're relaxed, you're not tense. When you tense your muscles and then relax them, you're learning what *not* to do—to not be tense. This way, you develop a sense of your muscles and what they're doing. Therapists have had positive results using Progressive Relaxation in treating anxiety, depression, insomnia, fatigue, mild phobias, and general muscle tension.

One reason you push yourself to be constantly busy is to avoid certain feelings and bodily sensations such as hunger pangs, muscle strain, tired eyes, fatigue, depression, anxiety, anger, stress, or tension. When you learn to relax, you have time to tune in to your body and to listen to what it has to say. These messages will offer you guidance as to what you need to attend to.

Once you know how to relax, dealing with emotions and bodily sensations becomes easier. Becoming aware of your body helps you release a variety of emotions, allowing them to move through your body until they're gone. When you deny or ignore your feelings, they stack up. The Progressive Relaxation technique is one way to let them go. Instead of engaging in harmful eating behaviors, use this technique to deal with

---

[4] Jacobson, E. *Progressive Relaxation*. Chicago: The University of Chicago Press, Midway Reprint, 1974.

stress, tension, and unpleasant emotions. Relaxation can delay, prevent, or become a substitute for unhealthy eating behaviors.

> *James found himself eating when he was tense and stressed. Food was the only thing that seemed to relax him quickly and completely, until he began to worry about the effects of eating so much. Then he felt stressed and angry at himself for giving in to bingeing. Once James learned how to relax his body through Progressive Relaxation, he didn't reach for food nearly as often as he had in the past. It was mainly when he didn't make the time for relaxation that he found himself eating to ease his emotions and stresses.*

To assess how tense your body is, sit in a chair or lie on the floor and tune in to how you feel. Your muscles and emotions will tell you the degree of tension you're experiencing at that moment. If you're anxious or your mind is racing, or if your muscles are tight or you have a desire to jump up and get going—you're not relaxed. Progressive Relaxation will teach you how to counter tension and stress, two of the most common reasons for turning to food or starving yourself.

The method addresses five main areas of the body and their corresponding muscles: hands and arms, feet and legs, torso and back, head and neck, and whole body.

Basic Instructions: Identify the particular muscles or muscle groups that feel tense. Then lie down and tense each muscle group for seven to ten seconds. Relax for 25 to 30 seconds in between. Repeat up to five times. Keep your eyes closed and focus on one muscle group at a time. As each muscle group is tensed then relaxed, imagine throwing that tension away, seeing it leave your body, or blowing it out with each breath.

1. Hands and Arms: Bend your elbow and tense your biceps in the left arm. Hold tightly, then relax and straighten your arm. Clench your left fist tighter and tighter to tense your triceps. Hold the clenched fist and study the tension in your fist, hand, and forearms. Let go and relax the arm. Now hold your arm straight down by your side and bend your hand back, then release. Stretch your straightened right arm across the front of your body, hold, and let go. Notice the contrast between the left arm and right arm. Now do the same thing with your right biceps, triceps, hand flexor, and shoulder socket, noticing the contrast between the sensations of relaxation and those of tension. Repeat the above procedure at least once.

2. Feet and Legs: Tense your left foot by pulling your toes back toward your head. Hold and then release. Now point your left toes, hold, and let go. Tense your left leg by pressing the heal downward. Feel the tension by holding this position, then release. Notice the contrast between your left leg and right leg. Do the same with your right foot and leg.

Notice the contrast between tension and relaxation, and any differences between your right side and left side. Repeat at least once.

3. Torso and Back: Draw in your stomach muscles, hold, then let go. Breathe in, filling your lungs completely—hold your breath and release it. Repeat inhaling, holding, and releasing your breath. Notice where your tension is located. Now arch your back, without creating strain and hold. Then place your back gently on the floor. Squeeze your shoulder blades together, hold, and release. Notice the difference between relaxation and tension.

4. Head and Neck: Observe any tension in your head or neck. Elevate your shoulders as if you're shrugging them, hold the position and release. Then, move your head in four directions, again holding it, then letting go: to the right, to the left, down towards your chest and up toward the top of your head. Wrinkle your forehead, holding it, then letting go. Now frown, letting the strain spread, then release, allowing your face to become smooth again. Close your eyes tightly. While they're closed, slowly turn your eyes toward the right, left, up, down, straight ahead, and then let go. Smile, hold the position, and release. Form your mouth into an "O" shape, hold, and let go. Stick out your tongue, hold it, then pull it back in, hold, and release. Clench your jaw, biting down. Feel the tension throughout your head, then let it go. Notice the difference between the tense state and the relaxed state. Your shoulders, head, forehead, eyes, mouth, tongue, and jaw are now relaxed. Notice how you feel. Repeat at least once.

5. Whole Body: Stretch your body, lifting your arms above your head and pointing your toes. Hold this position, then release it. Notice the difference between a previously tense body and a relaxed one. Follow your body from head to toes. Be in your body sensations. Feel the relaxation. Pay attention to the areas that feel very relaxed and the areas where it was harder to release the tension. Lie for a few minutes on the floor, relaxing.

Assignment: Do this relaxation technique one or two times a day or as often as necessary to be in touch with your body. You'll retrain yourself to tune in to and deal with any tension that arises.

3 - 10

Visualizations That Alter Beliefs:
Stop the Past From Haunting You

Visualizations are powerful tools to help you change aspects of your life that aren't working for you. Stopping the past from haunting you is just one effective use of visualizations. This chapter provides three visualizations to help you deal with negative beliefs that were formed in your childhood and adolescence. Once you heal the past, then you can live more fully in the present—viewing the world through more positive and realistic beliefs.

As I mentioned before, your beliefs shape and create your current reality. So as your beliefs change, so will your experiences. They can't help but be different. You cannot change the actual events that happened in the past, however, you can change your beliefs, which affect how you feel and think about yourself, and the decisions you make.

Give yourself the opportunity to understand what drives you to do the things you do. Once you can see the power of your beliefs, you'll want to develop new beliefs that promote health and well-being. These visualizations give you that opportunity. Use them as often as you need. They'll help you alter the beliefs that get in the way of you feeling good about yourself.

Assignment: When you're ready to work on your negative belief system at the belief level, choose one visualization technique with which to work. Each visualization is helpful in altering beliefs, although each has a slightly different focus. You can use these techniques as often as needed.

Visualization 1
Shame and Pain:
Heal What Wounds You

One of the most powerful ways to alter your belief system is to address the situations in which the negative beliefs developed. To do this, go back to those situations in childhood and adolescence that you experienced as wounding and imagine a different outcome.

"The actual situation can never be changed, however,
you can create a different ending in your mind."

It's important to work with these memories because they are what led to the beliefs you currently hold in your subconscious about yourself. Many wounding experiences have similar themes, therefore, by healing one, you touch the others. The actual situation can never be changed, obviously, since it has already occurred. However, you can create a different ending in your mind.

As I stated earlier, woundings are most often associated with being shamed.[5] Some shame is necessary for children to become conscientious, responsible adults, but when shaming is extreme or inappropriate, it causes woundings. Many parents don't intentionally inflict harm upon their children, yet children still become wounded. Parents generally want their children to grow up to be able to take care of themselves. However, the way they go about it can feel wounding to a child or adolescent. Some parents intentionally try to hurt their child, which can make the wounding experience all the more painful. Ultimately, however, how you perceive the event is what matters. If the event left you feeling wounded, you were, whether or not the intention was to hurt you. Underneath the feelings of shame is pain. And that pain is what the infant, child, or adolescent felt during a wounding experience. The person feels the shame from then on, because the original pain seems too big to remember and feel.

Negative beliefs grow out of these situations for a number of reasons. First, differentiating between right and wrong becomes difficult. Anything about you that isn't perfect is wrong, and you develop a feeling of being permanently flawed. Second, you

---

[5] Much of the information and specific techniques on healing shame come from "Ending Shame, Part I: Infancy," "Ending Shame, Part II: Psychic Contracts of Pain (Childhood)," "Ending Shame, Part III: Those Adolescent Years," and "Ending Shame, Part IV: Adult Shame" Lazaris tapes, © 1990 Concept: Synergy and is used by permission.

allow yourself few desires or passions because being perfect and in control are more important. Third, all your selves are somewhat separate, with their own issues and functions, which is why you can locate the child, the adolescent, the critic, and the healer. Fourth, within the original shaming experience there was pain.

"The way to release shame is to go back to the shaming situation, visualize it, then give it back to the people who gave it to you in the first place."

Sometimes it feels as if your spirit has been crushed, and in a way it has been. Some pain is part of growing up. Too much pain, though, imprisons the self, and the connection with your soul or spirit is lost. You cannot hear the messages from the deepest part of you that has answers to why you're going through what you are. Without having a relationship with your soul or spirit, you miss the profound meaning of your pain and are unable to place it in the context of the development of your soul. Emotional and physical pain is often the voice of your soul clamoring to be heard. When you listen, you create the opportunity to reconnect with your soul and heal your pain. The root of negativity is pain, so the pain needs to be healed to free yourself from a negative point of view. Shame creates feelings of guilt, which cover up the early feelings of pain. Shame and guilt are easier to feel than the original pain. As an adult, shame is often unconsciously passed on to others. This is done with the hope of getting rid of one's own shame, so as to never feel it again. However, it doesn't work. The way to release shame is to go back to the shaming situation, visualize it, then give it back to the people who gave it to you in the first place (your parents or other significant persons).

When you return shame, you reexperience the original pain. You process and release the feelings in the visualization through crying, yelling, screaming, kicking, and throwing things. You do this in your imagination, feeling whatever comes up and seeing yourself express your feelings. Processing your feelings by doing it this way can release years of pain without needing to confront your parents. This works well if your parents are no longer living, if they would be nonresponsive or hostile, or if it would hurt them too deeply to be dealt with directly. You have an opportunity to express the anger you have felt for a very long time but have been unable to release. Many beliefs and attitudes can be given back (e.g., perfectionism, control, martyrdom, body hate, or judgmental and critical attitudes). A number of wounding experiences have similar themes. So when you heal one, the others are touched. For that theme, you may only need to use the visualization a few times. Because feelings come in waves, you can use this technique when you recognize a negative belief that's creating problems.

Part of you will resist the change. Understand that resistance is a reaction to making changes. Acknowledge it, but don't let it detract from the work you're doing. The critic can become very frightened when he or she senses the possibility of change. Fears can get stirred up, and you can imagine all the horrible things that could happen. Generally, these fears don't materialize; they are a smoke screen to stop you from doing work that will lead you into unknown territory. At least with your old negative beliefs operating, life is predictable. Change leads to being in the scary unknown, which eventually becomes known.

Before starting the visualization to alter your beliefs and heal shame, explore and understand what situations in childhood and adolescence felt wounding and which negative beliefs developed as a result. It may take introspection to discover what happened and when. Do the groundwork prior to using this visualization.

You may want to do the visualization with a therapist or supportive friend, since it can feel frightening to give back something to your parents or significant persons that you've been holding on to for a long time. *You* decide everything that will happen in the visualization and *you* determine the outcome you're seeking, so there are no surprises. Do this technique when you're emotionally ready. There's no rush; you have the rest of your life to heal. You will know when you're ready to try. The healer within will let you know.

Giving Back Shame

1. Sit in a comfortable chair and take a few deep breaths. Imagine being in a safe place. Everyone has a place in their mind's eye that feels utterly safe. This may be in the mountains, by the water, in a meadow, or in a room of your favorite house. Once you're there, open all your senses to the surroundings. See the color of the sky, trees, grass, flowers, and water. Hear the rustling of leaves, water over rocks, birds singing. Smell the fragrance of flowers, the wet grass. Touch the roughness of bark, the coolness of water, the softness of flower petals. Taste the air.

2. When you're ready, go back to the experience you considered wounding. Imagine the situation unfolding across from where you are. Remember what occurred at that time, and see it clearly—as if it's happening to you right now. Recreate the events so it feels as if it's being played out all over again. See the room, notice the furniture and decor, and pay attention to what everyone is wearing, how they're acting, and what they're saying. Remember as many details as you can—it makes it more real. You already survived the situation, so you can survive revisiting the memory of it. Now, become the infant, child, or adolescent who was shamed. And notice how you decided all of this was your fault.

3. Feel how you felt about it then, as the situation unfolds. Experience whatever is there: fear, anger, sadness, anxiety, rage, loneliness, helplessness, hopelessness…all of it. Allow yourself to experience the feelings to their fullest intensity. Don't yo-yo in and out of the feelings. Let the "young" you experience the original feelings for as long as needed.

4. Step out of the young you and become the adult you. Stop the shaming by rescuing the young one. Stand in front of the young one and halt the parent's or significant person's actions by expressing how the adult part of you feels about this. Tell the person that you're stopping the abuse right now. The young you is experiencing the situation as abusive, and you're halting the action. Usually, anger comes up. Express the anger by talking, yelling, screaming, stomping up and down, or throwing objects. The parent or significant person will attend to everything you have to say—it's your visualization. Defend the young you. Show that you are your champion. Express your feelings until they're released and there is nothing else to say. Again, don't fluctuate in and out of the feelings. Experience and express the full intensity until you're done.

5. Take the young you away from the situation to a safe place and explain what has happened. Tell "yourself" what your parent or the significant person was doing—giving over his or her own shame because he or she didn't know what to do with it. The way the person was dealing with his or her shame was to pass it on to you in an abusive and unacceptable manner.

6. Let the young you express all the feelings that are present. The adult needs to listen without judgment or minimization. Be compassionate and understanding; assure the younger you that whatever he or she feels is absolutely fine. Hold, encourage, and help the young you through the emotions. Give whatever support is needed.

7. Explain to the young you that your parent or the significant person needs to be forgiven. Forgive the person for *why* he or she did it, not for *what* he or she did. The person did it because he or she was unconsciously passing on personal shame and unresolved issues from his or her past, not knowing any other way to get rid of them. That is the "why." You may not be able to forgive "what" they did—which felt abusive, and that's okay.

8. Forgive yourself for accepting the shame and negative beliefs. The young you didn't know any better.

9. Give back all the shame. Use a container of any kind, making sure it's large enough to hold it all. Put the shame in the container. Shame has a variety of forms and may look like many things. It may be words, papers, goo slipping off the body, bubbles coming from inside the body, or bundles of thoughts that pop out of the head. Use any form that comes to mind. Once the container is full and the lid is closed, help the young you walk back into the situation and hand it over to your parent or the significant person who accepts it.

10. After you give back the shame, walk away from the scene with the young you. Take the young one to a safe place and offer assurances that you are available whenever needed. The young you just needs to call and the adult will come.

11. When you're done, come out of the visualization. Sit quietly for a few moments. Wipe your eyes if you've been crying. Give yourself time to process what has happened. Be aware of the resistant part that doesn't believe this created any change. And let the work you just did be real.

Use this visualization as many times as necessary to heal shame and pain, and to change beliefs and attitudes. You can use this technique with any memory in which something was passed on to you and you no longer want it influencing your life to the degree it has been. Many situations outside the family experience can be shaming as well. This visualization will also work with those incidents.

Notice over time how the negative beliefs and shame tied to the memories you worked on are weaker and how your critic is quieter.

Visualization 2
In Your Room of Beliefs:
Replace Old Beliefs With New Ones

Another way to alter beliefs is to change them directly in your "Room of Beliefs."[6] Beliefs are imprinted in the brain, and we access them automatically. To get rid of one, we must replace it with a new one. This visualization will aid in replacing your old, outdated beliefs with healthier ones. Get to know what your beliefs are. If you're having trouble figuring out your beliefs, look at what's happening in your life that you dislike, and ask yourself, "What would a person have to believe to create this situation?" Your answer will offer clues to your beliefs. Once you decide which one you want to change, think about how you say the belief to yourself. Write it down on a piece of paper exactly as you say it in your head. Keep it simple. Then write the belief you want in the same syntax and sentence structure as the old belief. For example, you may believe "I am unlovable." Write down the new belief as "I am lovable." Once you've written the new belief, use it to replace the old one. When you're ready, follow the steps below. Get involved in the visualization by opening up all your senses. Be imaginative and get into the emotion of it.

Replacing a Belief

1. Sit in a comfortable chair and imagine being in your safe place. Once you're there, open up all your senses to the experience. See the color of the ocean, sky, meadow, trees, and hills. Hear the sounds of waves on the shore, wind in the trees, squirrels chewing nuts. Smell the fragrance of wet sand and seaweed. Touch the velvet of sand, the prickle of grass. Taste the air.

2. Once your senses are fully opened to the experience, walk toward the door. The door can be in the knot of a tree, on the side of a hill, a manhole in the grass, or any other likely or unlikely place. Open up the door and walk down the stairs into a basement—symbolically into your subconscious. It's a dark, dank, dusty, gray room filled with cobwebs—not scary, just old. Experience the room as you enter it. Notice what it looks like and how it feels to be there. As you walk across the basement, notice fragments from your past, such as a special toy or a report card (these will give you clues as to the

---

6 The "Room of Beliefs" technique may be found on "Discovering Your Subconscious" or "Secrets to Changing Anything in Your Life—Instantly" Lazaris tapes, © 1992 Concept: Synergy and is used by permission.

period in time when you learned this belief). Cross the room until you reach a red door. A sign on the door reads, "Room of Beliefs." Walk into the room, which is filled with brilliant, white light.

3.   Walk across the room to the table with the leather-bound book on top. The book's title is "My Beliefs and Attitudes." This is your own book of beliefs that you've been compiling since infancy. Open the book to the page with the belief written on it that you want to change. Read it to make sure that you have the right belief. Destroy the belief in three ways: rip the page out of the book; then pick up the black marker resting next to the book and write VOID in big black letters across the belief; finally, tear it into tiny pieces, and set them on fire. Burn them until there's nothing left but ashes, and scatter them. Once you've burned the paper, check the floor and your hands and clothing to make sure you haven't missed any pieces. If you have, burn those too. Once this is done, write the new belief on a blank page with the black marker. As you do so, sense yourself writing every letter, then look at it. When you're finished, close the book. You're done! Exit your "Room of Beliefs," walk through the basement room, up the stairs, and back into your safe place. Stay in your safe place as long as you need to, then open your eyes. Desire it, imagine it, and expect it to be different.

To reinforce the new belief, take an index card and write the new belief on it. Post it on the bathroom mirror. Every time you see it, say the belief to yourself in the mirror. Take another index card and cut it into small pieces. Write the belief on all the pieces and tape them to frequently seen places such as your alarm clock, rear view mirror, and refrigerator. As you say the belief to yourself, your subconscious will pick it up.

There will be a part of you that won't believe what you did will effect any real change. Listen to this part, acknowledge the message, and allow what you did to be real. You may not notice a difference right away. However, over time a subtle shift in thinking will catch your attention. If the belief is different, your thoughts and feelings will be different, and so will your behaviors, responses, decisions, and choices. They will correspond to the new belief.

You can use this visualization with any belief. It's a nice accompaniment to the first visualization, where you gave back the shame. Once the shame is returned, there's room for new beliefs.

Visualization 3
One Fell Swoop:
Give Back Negative Beliefs All at Once

Another method of giving back shame, negative beliefs, and unhealthy attitudes is to return them all in one fell swoop to the person who gave them to you in the first place. Family members and other adults who influenced you during your childhood and adolescence are the ones who shaped your beliefs and attitudes. You received both positive and negative beliefs. The positive beliefs are the ones you want to retain, plus you want to add more of them. Therefore, returning the negative beliefs to their rightful owners creates a space for healthier, more balanced beliefs and attitudes. Decide first what you're going to give back. For instance, you may want to give back your series of beliefs on having to be perfect. Determine to whom you're going to return them. Then you're ready for the next steps.

Giving It All Back

1. Stand or sit in a comfortable position. Surround yourself with white light. Think about the belief you no longer want to have. Shut your eyes and see the person who gave you the belief standing in front of you.

2. Cup both of your hands as if you're going to scoop up water from a stream to drink. Place your cupped hands behind your back, waist high, with the cupped part facing your back. Scrape your cupped hands around your body as if you're gathering something off your waist. You are gathering the "energy" attached to the beliefs that are connected to you. When you come to the front of your body, you will have in your cupped hands the belief, symbolically held.

3. With your eyes shut, see the person to whom you are returning the belief. Say to him or her, "I give you back to you," pushing your cupped hands out and toward the person, as if you are releasing a bird. Repeat this five to six times, one after the other.

You can do this visualization many times a day because it takes only a few seconds. Over time, you will begin to notice a subtle shift in the belief. It won't hit you over the head, but it will change ever so slightly, yet significantly.

WHERE YOU ARE NOW

By the end of **Part Three: Healing the Emotional Self and the Mental Self**, you'll understand your personal set of beliefs, attitudes, thoughts, and feelings, and how they affect the choices you make. You'll have the tools to change negative beliefs, alter critical internal dialogue, rid yourself of perfectionism, act more assertively, and become more of who you are. At the same time, you'll continue to work on developing healthier eating and exercise habits, and on accepting yourself the way you are. If you desire, go back to the areas you want to explore more fully. Check (✓) the areas you've completed.

_____ You've made the link between your belief system, the feelings you have, the thoughts you think, and the choices you make.

_____ You've defined your belief system and the attitudes you hold about yourself and others, linking your history with present-day interpretation of life events.

_____ You've explored why you turn to or deny yourself food. You see that what you do with food and the importance you place on weight and appearance are symptoms of something deeper.

_____ You've met your internal critic and are aware of the harsh messages your critic uses to reinforce negative beliefs.

_____ You've met your child and adolescent and can identify one or two experiences in which you felt shame and pain. You're able to link these events to negative beliefs and attitudes you hold, as well as to how you think and feel about yourself, others, and the world in general.

_____ You can hear the gentle voice of your healer, who encourages you to take care of and be kind to yourself.

_____ You've identified your personal set of negative beliefs.

_____ You've explored your thoughts and feelings that correspond to your beliefs.

_____ You've discovered the ways you engage in distorted thinking and how these distortions get played out in your life.

_____ You're actively refuting your critical internal voice whenever you catch yourself making critical self-statements.

_____ You've explored where, when, and how you strive for perfection, and how that makes you reject your perceived flaws.

_____ You're aware of when and with whom you compare yourself and catch yourself doing so.

_____ You've made a list of your strengths and flaws and are making accepting self-statements to accept all your characteristics.

_____ You're aware of where, when, and with whom you monitor your behaviors—or wear a mask—to fit a situation. You're taking steps to be your true, authentic self and to experience any feelings that arise when doing so.

_____ You're learning to become assertive in your communications with others.

_____ You're noticing when you're living in anticipation and what parts of yourself you're rejecting. You're making a conscious effort to fully experience each moment and to accept whatever happens in that moment.

_____ You're making self-affirmations daily on the aspects of yourself you want to accept, in an effort to chip away at negative beliefs and quiet the critic.

_____ You've tried Progressive Relaxation and have experienced the benefits of reducing stress and feeling relaxed.

_____ You've used one or more of the visualizations to alter negative beliefs, and you're developing more positive and realistic beliefs.

_____ You're continuing to plan and eat three meals a day, make healthier food choices, exercise moderately, reduce body hate, attend to your emotions, and cope with stressful events in ways other than turning to food.

_____ You're seeing results with weight loss if you're overweight, weight gain if you're underweight, and healthy self-acceptance if your body is staying the same.

With all the information you now have about your emotional self and mental self and the changes you've made, you're ready to move on to **Part Four: Healing the Spiritual Self.**

PART FOUR: HEALING THE SPIRITUAL SELF

4 - 1

Tending to the Soul: Find Your Way Back Home

In our modern-day, technologically advanced world, the concept of the soul seems to have all but disappeared. We demand facts, figures, and proof that something actually exists before we're willing to believe in it. But the soul is amorphous, and impossible to locate with scientific, research-oriented methods and tools. To believe in the soul is to believe in something more—more than what science can prove tangible or, in its terms, real.

"We as a culture have disowned the soul. Yet the soul is at the very center of our lives."

So what is the soul? It is the principle of life, feeling, and action in every human being; a distinct entity separate from the physical body; a spiritual part of humans that lies midpoint between understanding (consciousness) and unconsciousness. Because we cannot see it, feel it, or pinpoint its location or purpose, we doubt its existence. We as a culture have disowned the soul. Yet the soul is at the very center of our lives.

Whenever we disown something, it clamors to be noticed. When we're beset by emotional issues and uncomfortable physical sensations, it's often the voice of our soul yearning to be heard. Many people report chronic feelings of meaninglessness, emptiness, depression, and anxiety. They feel they've lost a sense of personal values, and they hunger for spirituality. They've simply lost connection with the soul. Material things and external achievements cannot replace this connection; they're not a cure for emptiness. In fact, they offer only a temporary sense of fulfillment, as many people who have attained these things can attest.

The drive for perfection is equally empty. It never brings the happiness we hope it will. Yet, our culture persists in believing that attaining perfection and material wealth will solve all of life's problems. But the key to reducing those painful feelings is turning inward (toward the soul) and upward (toward God or Goddess). This places emotions in context and gives the soul a voice.

Tending to the soul means tending to all your emotional and physical sensations with respect and awe; it means refusing to ignore or disown what you perceive as flaws. It's like tending a garden. You till the soil, plant the seeds, watch the plants grow, weed, water, fertilize, and enjoy the process. Do the same with your emotions—observe what you're feeling, what stirred up the feeling, what beliefs are behind it, and what you must do to process the feeling. During all this, own the feeling with great regard. Work with what's there, don't wish it to be different. When you honor your pain and go into it, rather than sidestepping it, a richness of experience develops, and you release the pain.

When you buy into the idea of a universal "normal" that you must achieve, you deprive yourself of a very personal connection with your soul. Your experiences are going to be different from anybody else's. That's why I highly recommend identifying your feelings, writing and talking about them, and sitting through the experience.

"Any wish for a simple, perfect, and consistently happy life is unrealistic and unattainable."

Pay attention to your emotional self, and you'll observe how the soul manifests itself and operates. Listen, and you'll hear your soul telling you that you need to pay attention and look inward. You need to observe and respect your emotions, rather than remove them. Process—yes, remove—no.

The tapestry of life is complex, just as the soul is. Any wish for a simple, perfect, and consistently happy life is unrealistic and unattainable. We all grow and change through our emotional experiences, not our mental exercises. Scientists can build computers to simulate mental processes and functions, but these machines can never feel. And it's that capacity to feel that makes humans special.

As you consciously watch your emotional life unfold, you'll catch glimpses into your soul. Tending to the soul also means attending to the small details of your everyday life—giving them meaning and value, thereby creating a depth of experience. It takes a daily, sometimes moment-to-moment commitment to respect and honor whatever emotional or physical experiences you have. This means paying attention to them, going through them, and coming out the other side knowing you've made it.

The Dark Side

We all have a shadow or dark side—those emotions and characteristics we perceive as flawed, and, therefore, intolerable. Since everyone has a dark side, it only becomes problematic when you disown your flaws because you are more likely to unconsciously act out your unresolved issues, feeling controlled by them. It's as if those aspects of the self have a life of their own, and the only way to control them is to ban them from your conscious awareness.

Yet painful emotional experiences and all your unique characteristics add richness to what otherwise would be a dull and predictable life. If you had only pleasurable experiences and positive traits, you'd be one-dimensional and boring. The depth of life comes from its duality—the light side and the dark side of the self. The dark side often provides the path to the light. By becoming consciously attuned to your flaws and owning them, you can then begin to make changes in behaviors you no longer want to exhibit. When you go through the dark, you learn to appreciate the light. This is what healing is all about. To create change, you can't go around the pain, using avoidance or denial, you must go through it. Once you can own your unpleasant emotional experiences and be with them, they change, move on, and dissipate. In that very experience, you connect with the deepest part of you.

Tending to the soul means accepting whatever feelings arise. Judgment stops the process. You'll feel no empathy or desire for exploration if you're judging each situation as bad or wrong. When you judge, you effectively block the path to the soul. Be with yourself and learn who you are in all your complexity. This kind of acceptance makes the painful experiences of life easier. Everybody has pain; it's what you do with it that counts. Honor it, feel it, allow yourself to move through it, and learn from it.

Each of your selves is an aspect of your soul. You're all the ages you have ever been, and being in touch with all your selves is part of being human. Tending to the soul means being in the present fully and completely. Problems arise when you continually live in the past and are unable to process it and let it go. But all you really have is the moment…not the future and not the past. By living each moment, your life becomes richer no matter what's happening at that time. This doesn't mean, however, that the present will always be pleasant, but it will be profound. Let your life be profound and meaningful. It's the only life you have.

Develop Your Spirituality

Tending to your soul means developing your spirituality and having a sense that there's something bigger than you in the universe, and you're a part of it. You'll discover a feeling that you're not alone in your existence, but are connected to a larger whole. So when you face pain, you'll feel reassured that you don't have to go it alone. When you ask for help or guidance, it's there for you. You access it through meditation, prayer, quiet contemplation, and by asking directly.

When infants come into the world, they're very connected to their souls. As time goes on and social conditioning occurs, they lose touch with and become alienated from their souls. Then they spend the rest of their lives trying to reconnect with their souls. That's what spirituality is all about—finding your way back home—or discovering the divine within you. Following that path involves giving up the idealized self, the self you want to be that embodies all the good qualities you strive to have and to show the world.

Once you can own all of you and live in the moment, you have tapped in to your soul and spirituality. It takes a daily commitment to stay on your unique spiritual path, wherever that may take you. And it means trusting that you have everything you need to change, grow, and be who you are—filled with self-acceptance, confidence, esteem, and worth. You'll no longer need food to fill the void, replacing it with a meaningful and magical connection with the deepest part of you.

Assignment: Now is the time to focus on your spiritual self and begin to tend to your soul. Take time to think about and feel what soul and spirit mean to you. Find ways to discover and express your spirituality. This is a very personal process. Each person's idea differs from everyone else's, so let your unique path unfold.

WHERE YOU ARE NOW

By the end of **Part Four: Healing the Spiritual Self,** you'll be connected more with your soul, understand your dark side and how you express this aspect of yourself, and begin to develop your own unique sense of spirituality. If you need to, go back to the areas you want to explore more fully. Check (✓) the areas you've completed.

_____ You're exploring what "soul" means to you. You're seeing that your feelings and physical sensations are often a message from your soul, nudging you to respectfully attend to these experiences.

_____ You're looking at your dark side—those very aspects of your character you deem unacceptable and bad—and are allowing yourself to experience your dark side along with your light side.

_____ You're defining what spirituality means to you and are exploring how you develop your own sense of what that is.

_____ You're continuing to address your emotional self and mental self by focusing on the issues you need to work through. You're making healthy changes in your belief system, thought processes, emotional reactions, and choices.

_____ You're also focusing on planning meals and eating three meals a day.

With all the information you now have about your spiritual self and the way you're defining your unique spiritual path, you're ready to move on to **Part Five: Conclusion.**

PART FIVE:
CONCLUSION

5 - 1

On the Path to Recovery:
What You Can Do to Continue the Healing Process

You can continue your healing and growth process in a number of ways. Just remember, you must address your physical, emotional, mental, and spiritual selves each day. Continue to use the techniques from this workbook that you found helpful. Below are some additional ways to address your whole being:

1. Meditation: The many forms and disciplines of meditation include Hatha Yoga, Kundalini Yoga, prayer, Transcendental Meditation, and various kinds of mantra meditations. Meditation offers deep relaxation and a path to peak or spiritual experiences. No one method is superior to another. All methods work on the same principle of quieting the inner noise or turmoil and connecting you with your many selves and with your soul. Explore different methods to find the ones most appropriate for you.

"Learning to soothe yourself is very important."

---

2. Visualizations: In addition to altering negative beliefs and healing shame, you can use visualizations to create change in a number of areas. The Resource section lists various books that provide visualization techniques.

3. Self-Nurturing: Once you truly believe you are valuable, nurturing becomes easier than and even preferable to turning to food. Nurturing means being gentle with your body and emotions. Listening to what you need to comfort yourself becomes a habit, just as ignoring your needs has been. Nurturing means knowing when to stop eating, working, and running around. It means allowing yourself to relax. Learning to soothe yourself is very important. Soothing activities include long baths, lying on the beach, playing in water, lounging in nature, getting massages or facials, playing a musical instrument, daydreaming to the radio, watching sports on TV, spending time with people who are special, dancing, singing, laughing, crying, going to the symphony, listening to opera, or whatever else healthfully releases you from your daily routine.

4. Psychotherapy and Support Groups: Throughout the healing process, both kinds of counseling can facilitate change and offer needed support. The path of growth and self-discovery is sometimes long and difficult. Individual therapy needs to focus mainly on unhealthy eating behaviors and the underlying reasons you turn to or deny yourself food. Therefore, I advise finding a therapist who specializes in this area. Groups come in many forms, ranging from those facilitated by a trained therapist to self-help groups led by peers. A number of self-help groups exist that address every area of addiction. Organizations that can help you find a therapist, group, or general information relevant to your healing process are listed in "Face Your Feelings: Alternatives to Feed Your Emotions," (chapter 2-15, p. 99).

Assignment: Follow any of the four suggestions to help you continue making the necessary changes within your physical, emotional, mental, and spiritual selves.

5 - 2

A New Lifestyle:
Maintaining the Positive Changes

Because unhealthy eating behaviors are used as a coping mechanism when you feel stressed, there's a possibility you'll return to the old familiar habits when you become stressed. To maintain the change you've worked for, become familiar with your specific trouble areas. Throughout this workbook, I've offered many strategies to help you deal with your eating patterns, negative beliefs, thoughts, feelings, and connections to your soul. Follow the steps below to maintain the positive changes you've made.

---

*"If your old behaviors begin to creep back in,
track the ones that have returned and
think about when and why they resurfaced."*

---

1. Monitor Behaviors: Begin by reflecting on the progress you've made. If your old behaviors begin to creep back in, track the ones that have returned and think about when and why they resurfaced. Identify your reasons for bingeing, grazing, purging, or starving by keeping a daily log of which stressful life events are leading to the eating behaviors. Sometimes, using the old behaviors to cope will seem a lot easier. If you find yourself falling back on old habits, work toward getting back on track as soon as possible.

2. Develop an Action Plan: Evaluate how you have been doing physically, emotionally, mentally, and spiritually the past month, week, and day. Review your action plan to determine whether or not it needs modifying. When you reevaluate your progress, key factors will emerge to show where your plan needs reinforcement. Assess which techniques in the workbook helped most in changing your behaviors, beliefs, thoughts, and feelings. Decide which of these would be the most useful at this point:

Addressing the physical self:

- Meal planning

- Distinguishing between physical or emotional hunger

- Incorporating "bad" foods

- Decreasing eating rituals

- Recognizing danger zones

- Delaying or preventing unhealthy behaviors

- Exercising appropriately

- Accepting your body

- Using alternative behaviors

Focusing on the emotional self and the mental self:

- Understanding negative beliefs

- Changing distorted thinking

- Ending perfectionism

- Decreasing the watchful eye

- Stopping nonassertive behaviors

- Ending living in the future

- Creating affirmations

- Inducing relaxation

- Working with visualizations

Addressing your spiritual self:

- Tending to your soul and fostering the development of your spirituality

Commit daily to working on those areas that are making you turn to the old eating patterns.

3. Process Feelings: Focus daily on your rich and complex emotional life. This includes assessing and identifying your feelings, accepting them as important messengers, processing them by sitting through them, journaling, talking with supportive people, or addressing the person or situation that has stirred up the feelings. When you don't process your feelings, you're more likely to turn to food to avoid or reduce the intensity of the emotional experience.

4. Plan Meals: Continue to plan what you will eat each day, and group foods into three separate meals. The ultimate goal is to eat regularly and moderately. When you become too restrictive with food, you're more likely to turn to bingeing or grazing to compensate for the food you've been denying yourself. Decide what you really want to eat and allow yourself to have it, within moderation.

5. Minimize Access to Binge Foods: When you're going through a particularly difficult time, don't keep food around that you would normally binge on. If you do, you'll be setting yourself up for failure. If you need to go food shopping, take precautions to not buy the binge foods: eat before you go to the store, take a limited amount of money, bring a grocery list, and buy only the foods that are on it.

"Eliminate thinness and perfection as measures of your acceptability."

---

6. Stop Weighing In: Unless there's a medical reason for weighing yourself regularly, such as anorexia or clinical obesity, stop using the scale as a measure of self-adequacy. Most likely you know what you weigh by how your clothes fit. When the number you see on the scale sets your daily mood, it's time to put the scale away. Besides, being overly concerned about your weight and shape is often due to other underlying feelings like depression or anxiety. Your body becomes an easy target for self-hatred and dissatisfaction. Work on the core issues instead of trying to change your body by taking extreme measures.

7. Develop Body Acceptance: One main reason people try to lose weight is so they'll like themselves. Regardless of what you weigh, you need a sense that the whole you is acceptable just the way it is. So eliminate thinness and perfection as measures of your acceptability. By doing this, you'll create a win-win situation. You win if you lose weight, you win if you don't. Either way, your body is acceptable and you'll feel better in general.

8. Exercise Moderately: Exercise can create a great sense of well-being. Moderate and regular exercise provides a variety of benefits: you'll reduce your stress, enhance your self-esteem, manage your weight better, and be able to relax.

9. Plan the Day's Events: Prevent unhealthy eating behaviors by planning activities that are incompatible with the old eating behaviors. You might meet with friends, exercise, get out of the house, take a bath or shower, brush your teeth, or try other diversions that come to mind. Create a list of three things you can do before turning to the familiar habits. Once you've done these alternatives, you're less likely to engage in bingeing, purging, starving, or grazing.

10. Set Realistic Goals: Set goals that are doable. If you create too many goals or they are too difficult, you're setting yourself up for disappointment. Focus on the smallest of changes, seeing them as successes. Most of us tend to label many experiences as "failures" and then see ourselves as failures. Monitor and acknowledge the areas in which you are making changes, even if they seem minute.

11. A New Lifestyle: All the changes you're making allow you to experience yourself and your life in a whole new way. You're giving yourself permission to be more fully involved and in touch with yourself. There's fear in changing, yet fear in staying the same. You're consciously choosing to make changes that will create a healthier way of life and you're accepting who you are in the process.

Assignment: Follow the eleven suggestions that will help you maintain the positive changes made up to now.

5 - 3

For the Family:
Ten Ways to Support a Loved One

Family members often don't know what to say or how to approach someone who's struggling with eating-disordered behaviors. These loved ones may mean well, however, their words and actions can be too intrusive or insensitive. Below are ten ways to support a loved one who's in the healing process. You may want to give this list to your family members.

"Eating disorders are not *a diet problem."*

---

1. Eating disorders are *not* a diet problem. They're complicated disorders related to the person's ability to identify, communicate, and cope with feelings and stressful life events.

2. You are not to blame. It's no one's "fault."

3. Do not encourage diets of any kind.

4. The goal of the person in recovery is to eat three balanced meals a day. This isn't your responsibility to enforce. Do not comment on foods eaten or not eaten. Don't hide food, force food on the person, or offer food to others but not to the person with the eating disorder.

5. Offer your support and convey the message that you're trying to understand their behaviors. Communicate that you will give support whenever it's asked for.

6. If you have any questions about the recovery process, ask directly. You'll receive information that's comfortable for the person to talk about. Do not push for more information, you'll end up with fewer answers, not more.

7. Do not tease, criticize, share opinions, or make judgments about weight, size, shape, or appearance. Saying nothing is better than making statements intended to change unhealthy behaviors.

8. Communicate your feelings directly. This may include any concerns regarding unhealthy eating habits and the healing process.

9. Be aware that one of the goals of healing is for the person to communicate more directly with you.

10. Understand that there's no immediate "cure." There are various stages of healing and many areas to address, which take time. The issues focused on during this process are many, and may resurface throughout healing.

Assignment: Family members don't always know how to deal with someone who struggles with food, weight, and body image. When you're ready, give this list to your family so they can understand how to approach you concerning your food issues.

5 - 4

Reap Success:
Keeping the Commitment to Change and Grow

You've made it! You have completed this workbook. What you asked yourself to do is change the way you deal with food, what you believe, and how you perceive yourself.

"Believe in yourself, even through the hardest of times—they don't stay difficult forever."

Quite a task from one short workbook. The successes you reap will come from continually working on these issues day by day. Make a commitment to yourself to create changes and continue to grow, and you'll gain a feeling of satisfaction. Making these changes is by no means comfortable or easy. It may be the hardest thing you ever do. However, you have it in you to redirect your life. Ultimately, the healing is up to you. Therapists, physicians, support groups, workshops, friends, and family members can be helpful. Seek the resources necessary for you to heal. Believe in yourself, even through the hardest of times—they don't stay difficult forever. When you work on yourself, you'll move forward and eventually find yourself at the place where you want to be—physically, emotionally, mentally, and spiritually. You can make the changes you desire! With time, energy, and commitment, you can become healthier and happier than you ever thought possible.

Assignment: Now that you've finished the workbook, see the successes you've created by making positive changes. If you need to, go back and work on areas that you want to refine and strengthen. Congratulate yourself for a job well done!

WHERE YOU ARE NOW

By the end of **Part Five: Conclusion,** you'll have made many important changes in your physical, emotional, mental, and spiritual selves. Check (✓) the areas you've completed.

You're developing a new style of eating you can use for the rest of your life. In doing so you're:

_____ planning and eating three meals a day

_____ making healthier food choices

_____ including the foods you love

_____ avoiding danger zones

_____ delaying or preventing unhealthy behaviors

_____ exercising appropriately

_____ accepting your body the way it is

_____ attending to your emotions

_____ using alternatives to food to cope with life's ups and downs

_____ reducing the time spent in relapse or in preventing an episode altogether

_____ losing weight if overweight, gaining weight if underweight, or staying the same—letting your body decide what's a healthy weight for you

You're eliminating the underlying reasons why you struggled with food, weight, and body-image. In doing so, you're:

_____ changing negative beliefs into more positive and realistic ones

_____ altering negative thoughts and feelings by balancing them with positive and neutral ones

_____ changing distorted thinking by refuting your critic

_____ reducing the harsh, judgmental internal dialogue

_____ increasing healthy self-talk

_____ developing self-acceptance, which enhances your self-esteem and worth

_____ reducing the drive for perfection by accepting strengths and flaws

_____ becoming more authentic by showing your true self

_____ living more in the moment and less in the future

_____ inducing relaxation and stress reduction on a regular basis

_____ reducing childhood and adolescent woundings by healing shame and pain

_____ becoming emotionally and mentally healthier overall

You're developing a connection with your soul and fostering your spirituality. In doing so, you're:

_____ creating a relationship with your soul

_____ understanding your dark and light side

_____ defining and developing your spirituality

You're focused on continuing the healing process. In doing so, you're:

_____ using any of the following that you find helpful—meditation, visualizations, self-nurturing techniques, and psychotherapy or support groups

_____ maintaining positive changes by doing such things as processing feelings, stopping weighing yourself, planning the day's events, and setting realistic goals

_____ providing family members with guidelines on how to approach you when they're concerned about your well-being

_____ allowing growth and change to create space for happiness and peace of mind

Congratulations! You've created a *Diet-Free Solution to Lifelong Weight Management*. Let the changes you've made be real and significant. You've put a lot of work into creating a new lifestyle for yourself. Continue to address the areas that need fine-tuning. Remember, you don't have to change everything all at once. Let the process unfold at a pace that's comfortable for you.

RESOURCES

American Anorexia/Bulimia Association (AA/BA)
293 Central Park West, Suite 1R
New York, NY 10024
(212) 501-8351

American Psychological Association (APA)
First Street, NE
Washington, D.C. 20002-4242
(202) 336-5500

Anorexia Nervosa and Related Eating Disorders (ANRED)
P.O. Box 5102
Eugene, Oregon 97405
(503) 344-1144

Concept: Synergy
P.O. Box 3285
Palm Beach, Florida 33480
(800) 678-2356

National Association of Anorexia Nervosa and Associated Disorders (ANAD)
Box 7
Highland Park, Illinois 60035
(847) 831-3438

National Eating Disorders Organization (NEDO)
Laureate Eating Disorder Program
6655 South Yale Avenue
Tulsa, Oklahoma 74136
(918) 481-4044

Overeaters Anonymous (OA)
6075 Zenith Court, NE
Rio Rancho, New Mexico 87124-6424
(505) 891-2664

Rational Recovery Systems (RRS)
P.O. Box 800
Lotus, CA 95651
(916) 621-4374

SEMINARS AND WORKSHOPS

Deirdra Price, Ph.D., is available for speaking engagements and training workshops. If your organization is interested in a presentation on *Healing the Hungry Self* or other topics related to lifelong weight management, please send inquiries to or call:

Deirdra Price, Ph.D.
President and CEO
Diet Free Solution
3555 Fourth Avenue
San Diego, CA 92103
(619) 491-9272
(800) 521-6067

WOULD YOU LIKE TO SHARE YOUR EXPERIENCES?

If you would like to share your experiences with *Diet Free Solution*, we would like to hear from you. We are interested in knowing how you are benefiting from *Healing the Hungry Self: The Diet-Free Solution to Lifelong Weight Management.* You can send the information anonymously if you wish. Please send information on the types of changes you made in your eating or exercising habits, how much weight you lost, how you're doing with accepting your body, how you're coping with your emotions, what beliefs you've changed, how distorted thinking affected your life, the ways you've let perfectionism go, and the connection you're developing with your soul and spirituality.

ORDER FORM

Please send me _____ (number of copies) of *Healing the Hungry Self: The Diet-Free Solution to Lifelong Weight Management* at a cost of $21.95 per copy plus shipping and handling.

BILL TO:

_____
Name

_____
Address

_____
City   State   Zip

_____
Phone (Day)

SHIP TO:

_____
Name

_____
Address

_____
City   State   Zip

_____
Phone (Day)

SHIPPING AND HANDLING CHARGES:

# of Items:	1	2	3	4	5
Book Rate: (2–4 weeks)	3.75	4.75	5.75	7.25	8.25
Priority: (3–5 days)	5.00	7.00	10.00	12.80	15.00

PAY BY CHECK OR CREDIT CARD:

○ Check   ○ Visa/Mastercard

_____ _____
Credit Card #   Expiration

_____
Signature

Diet Free Solution
3555 Fourth Avenue
San Diego, CA 92103

Order by Fax: (619) 435-0280

Or Call: (800) 521-6067

BOOK TOTAL $_____

CA DELIVERY (7.75% Sales Tax) $_____

SHIPPING/HANDLING $_____

TOTAL $_____

Prices are subject to change without notice.

REFERENCES

REFERENCES AND SUPPORTING RESEARCH

American Psychiatric Association. *Diagnostic and Statistical Manual of Mental Disorders* (4th Edition). Washington, D.C.: APA, 1994.

Brownell, K. and Rodin, J. The Dieting Maelstrom: Is It Possible and Advisable to Lose Weight? *American Psychologist, 49*:9, 1994.

Concept: Synergy. Lazaris Tapes. Palm Beach, Florida: NPN Publishing.
 Discovering Your Subconscious, 1986.
 Ending Shame, Part I: Infancy, 1990.
 Ending Shame, Part II: Psychic Contracts of Pain (Childhood), 1990.
 Ending Shame, Part III: Those Adolescent Years, 1990.
 Ending Shame, Part IV: Adult Shame, 1990.
 Giving Voice to Your Soul, 1993.
 Secrets to Changing Anything in Your Life—Instantly, 1992.
 The Secrets of Manifesting What You Want, Part I, 1986.

Davis, M., Eshelman, E., and McKay, M. *The Relaxation and Stress Reduction Workbook.* Oakland, California: New Harbinger Publications, 1988.

Garner, D. Dieting Maelstrom or Painful Evolution? *American Psychologist, 50*:11, 944–945, 1995.

Halmi, K. Changing Rates of Eating Disorders: What Does It Mean? *American Journal of Psychiatry, 152*:9, 1256–1257, 1995.

Harris Poll of 1,250 People. *American Health,* 6, 1995.

Horm, J. and Anderson, K. Who in America Is Trying to Lose Weight? *Annals of Internal Medicine, 119*:7, 672–676, 1993.

Institute for Natural Resources. *Mood, Mind, and Appetite Workshop,* 1995.

Jacobson, E. *Progressive Relaxation.* Chicago: The University of Chicago Press, Midway Reprint, 1974.

Johnson, C., and Flach, C. Characteristics of 105 Patients with Bulimia. *American Journal of Psychiatry, 142*:11, 1321–1324, 1985.

Kay, W., Weltzin, T., Hsu, L., McConaha, C., and Bolton, B. Amount of Calories Retained after Binge Eating and Vomiting. *American Journal of Psychiatry, 150*:6, 969–971, 1993.

McKay, M., and Fanning, P. *Self-Esteem: A Proven Program of Cognitive Techniques for Assessing, Improving, and Maintaining Self-Esteem.* Oakland, California: New Harbinger Publications, 1987.

National Association of Anorexia Nervosa and Associated Disorders. ANAD Ten Year Study, 1995.

Price, D. A Model of the Sense-of-Self in Normal Weight Bulimic Females. *Academic Dissertation,* California School of Professional Psychology, 1989.

Remington, D., Fisher, G., and Parent, E. *How to Lower Your Fat Thermostat.* Provo, Utah: Vitality House International, Inc., 1983.

Simon, J. *Conquering Heart Disease.* New York: Little, Brown, 1994.

Stice, E., and Shaw, H. Adverse Effects of the Media Portrayed Thin-Ideal on Women and Linkages to Bulimic Symptomology. *Journal of Social and Clinical Psychology, 13*:3, pp. 288–308, 1995.

Stunkard, A. and Penick, S. Behavior Modification in the Treatment of Obesity. *Archives of General Psychiatry, 36*:7, 1979.

SUGGESTED READINGS

Almaas, A. H. *Diamond Heart (Book Three): Being and the Meaning of Life.* Berkeley, California: Diamond Books, Almaas Publications, 1990.

Boskind-White, M., and White, W. C. *Bulimarexia: The Binge/Purge Cycle.* New York: W. W. Norton & Company, 1983.

Bradshaw, J. *Healing the Shame That Binds You.* Deerfield Beach, Florida: Health Communications, Inc., 1988.

Bruch, H. *The Golden Cage: The Enigma of Anorexia Nervosa.* New York: Random House, 1978.

Cauwels, J. M. *Bulimia: The Binge/Purge Compulsion.* New York: Doubleday & Company, 1983.

Chernin, K. *The Hungry Self: Women, Eating, and Identity.* New York: Harper & Row, 1985.

Fisher, S. *Discovering the Power of Self-Hypnosis: A New Approach for Enabling Change and Promoting Healing.* New York: Harper Collins, 1991.

Gawain, S. *Creative Visualizations.* New York: Bantam Books, 1978.

Gawain, S. *Living in the Light.* Mill Valley, California: Nataraj Publishing, 1986.

Hollis, J. *Fat Is a Family Affair.* San Francisco: Harper & Row, 1985.

Johnson, C., and Connors, M. *The Etiology and Treatment of Bulimia Nervosa: A Biopsychosocial Perspective.* New York: Basic Books, 1978.

Levenkron, S. *The Best Little Girl in the World.* New York: Warner Books, 1978.

Levenkron, S. *Treating and Overcoming Anorexia Nervosa.* New York: Warner Books, 1982.

McFarland, B., and Baker-Baumann, T. *Feeding the Empty Heart: Adult Children and Compulsive Eating.* San Francisco: Hazelden, 1989.

Miller, A. *The Drama of the Gifted Child.* New York: Basic Books, 1981.

Moore, T. *Care of the Soul.* New York: Harper Collins, 1994.

Orbach, S. *Fat Is a Feminist Issue.* New York: Berkeley Publishing, 1978.

Ross, R. *Prospering Women: A Complete Guide to Achieving the Full, Abundant Life.* New York: Bantam Books, 1982.

Roth, G. *Breaking Free From Compulsive Overeating.* New York: New American Library, 1984.

Roth, G. *Feeding the Hungry Heart: The Experience of Compulsive Eating.* New York: New American Library, 1982.

Sandbeck, T. *Deadly Diet: Recovering From Anorexia and Bulimia.* Oakland, California: New Harbinger, 1986.

Satir, V. *Meditations and Inspirations.* Berkeley, California: Celestial Arts, 1985.

Thesenga, S. *The Undefended Self: Living The Pathwork of Spiritual Wholeness.* Madison, Virginia: Pathwork Press, 1994.

Waterhouse, D. *Outsmarting the Female Fat Cell: The First Weight Control Program Designed Specifically for Women.* New York: Hyperion, 1993.

Whitfield, C. *Healing the Child Within.* Deerfield Beach, Florida: Health Communications, 1987.

Woodman, M. *Addiction to Perfection: The Still Unravished Bride.* Atrium Books, 1995.